Practical Binocular Vision Assessment

For Butterworth-Heinemann:

Publishing Director: Caroline Makepeace
Development Editor: Kim Benson
Project Manager: Ailsa Laing
Designer: George Ajayi
Illustrations Manager: Bruce Hogarth

Practical Binocular Vision Assessment

Frank Eperjesi BSc(Hons) PhD MCOptom DipOrth MILTHE

Lecturer and Research Optometrist, Neurosciences Research Institute,
School of Life and Health Sciences, Aston University, Birmingham, UK

Michelle M Rundström BSc(Hons) MCOptom DBO

Primary Care Optometrist and Sessional Orthoptist, Nottingham, UK

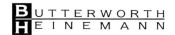

BUTTERWORTH
HEINEMANN

EDINBURGH LONDON NEW YORK OXFORD PHILADELPHIA ST LOUIS SYDNEY TORONTO 2004

BUTTERWORTH-HEINEMANN
An imprint of Elsevier Limited

First published 2004

ISBN 0 7506 5010 9

British Library Cataloguing in Publication Data
A catalogue record for this book is available from the British Library

Library of Congress Cataloging in Publication Data
A catalog record for this book is available from the Library of Congress

Notice
Medical knowledge is constantly changing. Standard safety precautions must be followed, but as new research and clinical experience
broaden our knowledge, changes in treatment and drug therapy may
become necessary or appropriate. Readers are advised to check the
most current product information provided by the manufacturer of
each drug to be administered to verify the recommended dose, the
method and duration of administration, and contraindications. It is
the responsibility of the practitioner, relying on experience and
knowledge of the patient, to determine dosages and the best
treatment for each individual patient. Neither the Publisher nor
the authors assumes any liability for any injury and/or damage to
persons or property arising from this publication.

The Publisher

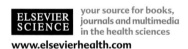

your source for books,
journals and multimedia
in the health sciences

www.elsevierhealth.com

The
publisher's
policy is to use
**paper manufactured
from sustainable forests**

Printed in China

Contents

Preface

Binocular vision assessment is often considered to be a confusing and challenging subject. Novices can become easily frustrated and lack confidence regarding clinically appropriate diagnosis. It is our view that difficulty in obtaining the correct diagnosis occurs as a consequence of inappropriate tests and inaccurate techniques.

We have attempted to remedy this by writing a guide to binocular vision assessment with a practical emphasis. The content is based on our understanding of current standard clinical practice, extensive experience of managing binocular vision problems, and teaching binocular vision at both undergraduate and postgraduate levels. We have not attempted to cover all aspects of binocular vision and this is certainly not a reference text. It is intended to be a simple step-by-step practical guide to assist the student and novice in developing and improving clinical techniques, to enable accurate diagnosis leading to successful management.

We would be grateful to receive any comments, positive or negative, via our publisher, so that we may be able to improve future editions of this book.

Frank Eperjesi/Michelle M Rundström
Birmingham/Nottingham, 2004

Acknowledgements

Thanks to Barry Brookes of Aston University for taking all the photographs, and to Rosie Auld and Clare Heath of the Birmingham and Midland Eye Centre for help in obtaining volunteers for the video clips, and Drs Fiona Baker, Sally Embleton and Ed Mallen for assistance with production of the video clips.

Introduction

One of our colleagues refers to binocular vision (BV) assessment as a 'black art', implying that anyone who has the slightest proficiency in dealing with patients who have binocular vision problems is a wizard or witch. Indeed, we have noticed that many eye-care practitioners express negativity when it comes to teaching or learning about BV anomalies and dealing with patients who have these problems.

While it is true that there are many BV anomalies that are difficult to diagnose and treat, these are found mainly in the Hospital Eye Service (HES) and are managed by orthoptists and ophthalmologists. Cases that an optometrist is likely to come across in primary care practice are usually easy to diagnose and (in certain cases) manage.

Correct diagnosis and management is more likely when attention is paid to the data-gathering process. By data-gathering we refer to the history and symptoms, vision and visual acuity measurement, cover test, oculomotility, refraction and other relevant tests (which are often incorrectly described as ancillary or supplementary), such as fusional reserves, stereoacuity, AC/A ratio and fixation disparity. Unfortunately, it is our experience that these procedures are often carried out inadequately or inaccurately, and therefore successful management becomes unlikely.

The equipment required to carry out a thorough BV assessment is simple and readily available: a cover stick, detailed near fixation targets, a pen torch with an on–off switch (see Fig. 3.1, p. 21), prism bars, RAF rule and distance and near Mallett units.

Binocular vision is a difficult subject to master just by listening to lectures and reading books – practical experience is essential. This often takes the form of observing and being supervised by an orthoptist or optometrist. However, making a diagnosis while observing a qualified practitioner is not as challenging as when examining a patient unaccompanied. Students express concern that all patients with BV anomalies are referred to the HES and it is difficult to access them. This is true to some extent, but there are many patients that present for routine refraction who have been discharged from the HES with heterophoria, fixation disparity and even long-standing heterotropia. Patients should not be categorized into those who attend for refraction and those who attend for a BV problem, because they are often one and the same. All routine refraction patients should be assessed by cover test, oculomotility and fixation disparity at least. Practice might not make perfect, but it certainly makes better.

The analogy that we use is learning to drive. In the early days novice drivers pay most attention to the mechanics of driving and less attention to where they are going. After a while, the procedure of driving becomes secondary and deciding where to go is the primary concern. The same is true for BV assessment. Initially, attention should be paid to the procedures, making sure that test target choices are appropriate and that working distances and positions are correct. With time, the procedures become more automatic and consequently it becomes easier to observe eye movements and concentrate on the diagnosis, and then management. This book is designed to facilitate proficiency with procedures and to allow the novice to reach the stage where diagnosis and management become the primary concern.

Our aim is to provide the novice eye-care practitioner encountering people with BV anomalies with a book that is sound, easy to read, relevant and of useful application. With this in mind, we have concentrated on investigation. For those readers wanting to gain a greater insight into other areas of BV, such as management, we can recommend the following books: Evans (2002) *Pickwell's Binocular Vision Anomalies*, 4th edn, and Evans & Doshi (2001) *Binocular Vision and Orthoptics: Investigation and Management*, both published by Butterworth-Heinemann.

We have learned from our own teaching experiences and have taken account of the difficulties that our own students have encountered when studying BV. For this reason we have chosen to limit the theoretical content of the book to a level that is sufficient for understanding the procedures involved, yet which does not overshadow the practicalities of their execution.

History and symptoms

Introduction

This part of the eye examination is extremely important. In the medical world it is frequently stated that 70% of diagnoses can be made from a good history and symptoms. Observations, such as a compensatory head posture (CHP), lid abnormalities and anisocoria, made at this stage of the examination can provide valuable clues to assist in the eventual diagnosis. We have found the following to be a useful framework in our clinical practice.

Paediatric cases

For children who seem nervous, it is best to start by conversing with a carer – usually but not always the mother – and to determine the main reason for the visit. Once the child has seen and heard a carer talking in a friendly manner, he or she may become less nervous; this will often help to improve cooperation during the examination. If the child is cooperative from the outset, once a few preliminary greetings are over the child can be addressed directly. It is important to discover in the child's own words whether he or she is having any vision or eye problems and, if so, what they are. We advocate noting the exact words the child uses to describe any visual problems. Sometimes information is obtained in this way that even the parent is unaware of. It is wise to corroborate all statements from children with a carer to check for accuracy. Of course, birth details, illnesses when the child was younger and family history questions will have to be asked directly of the carer. It is imperative that the main reason for the visit is determined and that this concern is addressed in the final summary. The main reason for attendance will also determine to a large extent the tests used during the examination.

The following questions can be asked of the child where possible, and confirmed by the carer where appropriate. However, taking the history and symptoms will vary according to the maturity of the child; the following list of questions is not meant to be exhaustive or prescriptive.

Young children (e.g. aged less than 4 years)

- Main reason for attending?
- Any near vision or distance vision concerns from the parents?
- Has a lazy eye been diagnosed?
- If problems exist, for how long have they been apparent?
- If these problems are long-standing, what was the age at onset?
- Is there current spectacle wear?
- From what age have glasses been used and what tasks were they recommended for?
- Have there been any previous HES visits?
- Any previous ocular trauma?

- Any previous patching?
- Any previous or current use of prisms?
- How is the current general health?
- Any family history of strabismus (eye turns), amblyopia (lazy eye), refractive correction (use of spectacles), eye operations?
- Were there any prenatal factors?
- What was the maternal age at birth?
- What was the maternal health at birth?
- Was there any toxaemia during the pregnancy?
- Were there any postnatal factors?
- Was there any fetal distress?
- Was the delivery assisted?
- Was the baby classed as premature?
- Was the baby small for dates?
- Was the birthweight low? (≤ 1500 g)

Any affirmative questions with respect to the birth history should heighten the index of suspicion. For example, it is known that one third of children born prematurely will have eye problems.

Older children

For older children who are able to respond directly to questioning, some questions will still need to be asked from the carer and most answers will need to be corroborated.

- Main reason for attending?
- Any near vision or distance vision concerns?
- Any headaches?
- Any eyestrain?
- Is there a lazy eye?
- If problems exist, for how long have they been apparent?
- If these problems are long-standing, what was the age at onset?
- Is there current spectacle wear?
- From what age have glasses been used and what tasks were they recommended for?
- Have there been any previous HES visits?
- Any previous ocular trauma?
- Any previous patching?
- Any previous orthoptic (eye) exercises?
- Any previous or current use of prisms?
- How is the current general health?
- Any family history of strabismus (eye turns), amblyopia (lazy eye), refractive correction (use of spectacles), eye operations?
- Were there any prenatal factors?
- What was the maternal age at birth?
- What was the maternal health at birth?
- Was there any toxaemia during the pregnancy?
- Were there any postnatal factors?
- Was there any fetal distress?
- Was the delivery assisted?
- Was the baby classed as premature?
- Was the baby small for dates?

- Was the birthweight low? (≤ 1500 g)
- Are there any current learning difficulties, especially with reading and writing?

Adults

- Main reason for attending?
- Any current vision or eye problems?
- Any near vision or distance vision concerns?
- Are you a keen reader? If not, is this through choice or is it related to your eyes?
- Any headaches?
- Any eyestrain?
- Any double vision?
- Is there a lazy eye or an eye that does not see as well as the other?
- If problems exist, for how long have they been apparent?
- If these problems are long-standing, what was the age at onset?
- Is there current spectacle wear?
- From what age have glasses been used and what tasks were they recommended for?
- Have there been any previous HES visits?
- Any previous ocular trauma?
- Any previous patching?
- Any previous orthoptic (eye) exercises?
- Any previous or current use of prisms?
- How is the current general health?
- Any family history of strabismus (eye turns), amblyopia (lazy eye), refractive correction (use of spectacles), eye operations?
- Any family medical history of glaucoma, cataract, age-related macular degeneration (wearing out of the eyes), hypertension (high blood pressure), diabetes (insulin dependent or non-insulin dependent), heart disease, thyroid problems?
- Family ocular history, strabismus, success of treatment, glasses
- General health
- Medication
- Any connection with current symptoms (e.g. change of occupation and VDU work)
- Birth history, full term, normal delivery, complications

Reason(s) for attending may include a general (routine) eye examination, change in visual acuity, headaches or diplopia:

- If the patient complains of headaches, it is important to ask about the frequency – whether they occur in the morning or later in the day; whether the headaches wake the patient during the night; their duration and onset.
- If diplopia is a presenting symptom, it is necessary to note whether it is recent or long-standing, the type (horizontal, vertical, torsional or a combination), whether it occurs at distance or near, or both, methods of overcoming the diplopia, mode of onset (sudden onset may mean a palsy, gradual onset may mean decompensation).
- Does it occur when looking to one side or up or down?
- Any idea what might have caused it?

Measurement of visual acuity

Introduction

In the field of eye care, vision is often described as the smallest symbol or letter that can be identified without the use of an optical device such as spectacles or contact lenses. Visual acuity can be described as the smallest symbol or letter that can be identified with the aid of an optical device such as spectacles or contact lenses. For reasons of simplicity and brevity only visual acuity is referred to in this chapter, but the reader should remember that vision and visual acuity are different entities.

Accurate assessment of visual acuity is important in terms of detecting and monitoring disease, determining the outcome of refraction, and choosing targets to use in cover testing (see Chapter 3). Tests that use letters or symbols (also known as optotypes) such as the Snellen chart, can be described as recognition or identification (minimum recognisable) charts. Tests that use preferential looking such as the Keeler acuity or Cardiff acuity cards, can be described as resolution (minimum resolvable) charts. All visual acuity charts record an estimate of the visual acuity; this depends on several factors including the visual acuity, motivation and attention of the patient, the presence of any pathology and the skill of the examiner.

For most young children, visual acuity should be measured with each eye in turn, and then binocularly; this will depend on cooperation. If there is some suspicion that one eye sees poorly – perhaps from a health visitor, school nurse or orthoptic screening referral letter – the suspect eye should be tested first.

Even young children are quite capable of remembering letters from one eye to the next, so different letters of approximately equal difficulty should be used for each visual acuity determination. For young children it is probably better to attempt a binocular near-visual acuity (to build confidence) measurement before going on to determine monocular near-visual acuity. Occlusion of a young child in order to carry out monocular visual acuity assessment is probably best achieved by sitting the child on the parent's lap and asking the parent to cover each eye in turn, taking care not to let the child peek between their fingers or to press too firmly, distort the cornea and lead to an artificially reduced visual acuity measurement when that eye is assessed. An alternative is to use a lightweight child's spectacle frame glazed with an occluder or frosted lens on one side. For older children it is better to use either a hand-held occluder such as a cover stick or an occluding trial lens placed in the trial frame.

There are several different types of visual acuity chart; perhaps the most commonly used are the standard 6-m Snellen chart with a mirror, the Sheridan–Gardiner test and the logMAR acuity test (also known as Keeler crowded cards); all can be used with or without matching cards. For many young children it is not possible to use the 6-m Snellen chart with a mirror, because the mirror may confuse them or they may just turn around and look directly at the chart.

Readers of this book are likely to be aware that single letters are easier to identify than letters arranged in groups; with single letters there is less contour interaction and the crowding phenomenon is reduced. However, practitioners may not have realized that pointing to one letter on a line of letters with a finger also reduces contour interaction and therefore makes the task easier than reading the line without pointing. Finger-pointing should be noted on the record card as a memo that the child did not achieve grouped-letter visual acuity.

All patients, no matter what their age, should be encouraged to guess letters, especially if they read a line of letters quickly and accurately, and then stop. Forcing patients to their visual acuity threshold will make the measurement more accurate (forced choice) as many patients will go on to read another line, or line and a half, quite well. Patients should be encouraged and allowed to guess, but not allowed to lean or move forward. For older people with visual acuity of less than 6/60 in one or both eyes, a single 6/60 letter printed on to white paper can be used to assess visual acuity. The practitioner can position the letter at the appropriate distance and measure visual acuity without asking the patient to move from their chair.

For more detailed information about the tests described below, the reader is referred to the instruction booklet that accompanies each test.

Distance visual acuity tests

Snellen chart

This was the first standardized visual acuity chart, developed in 1862. Probably the most widely used chart (Fig. 2.1), it is quick and easy to use, familiar to clinicians and patients worldwide, and correlates well with the patient's subjective visual acuity in most, but not all, cases. However, the Snellen chart does suffer from many well documented design problems:

- Some letters are easier to see than others, especially when small.
- The relative legibility of letters depends on the magnitude and axis of any uncorrected astigmatism.
- Many versions fail to adhere to the recommendations and standards relating to the selection of letters.
- Most charts have one 6/60 letter and an increasing number of letters on lower lines. Patients with poor visual acuity are required to read fewer letters than those with good visual acuity.
- The small number of large letters limits the chart's usefulness when assessing people with very poor visual acuity.
- Letters on lower lines are more crowded than those towards the top of the chart, and crowding increases the task difficulty so that the visual demand changes down the chart.
- The spacing between each letter and each row of letters bears no systematic relationship to the width and height of letters. For this reason visual acuity measured at a distance of less than 6 m cannot easily be converted to a 6-m equivalent.

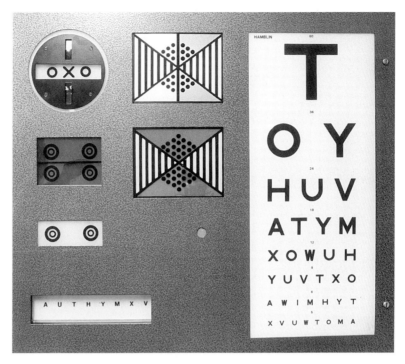

Fig. 2.1   *Snellen visual acuity chart.*

- Most Snellen charts are designed to be used with a mirror to provide a 6-m working distance; the concept of how a mirror works can be confusing for many young children.
- The progression of letter sizes follows an approximate geometrical progression, with letter size doubling every other line.
- Progression is irregular, with extra lines at the bottom and lines omitted at the top.
- Statistical analysis of results is precluded and therefore the chart has little use in modern eye-care research.
- Visual acuity is noted as the lowest line of letters read. In practice, patients seldom read all of one line and no letters on the line below, and sometimes the endpoint may spread over three lines; for example, the result 6/6 – 3 + 2 is difficult to convey and could easily be noted as 6/9 + 4 + 2. There are no agreed standards for this type of notation and there is ample room for confusion.
- Clues to active pathology can be missed; for example, a patient with a best corrected visual acuity of 6/7.5 will be measured as 6/9 because most Snellen charts do not have a 6/7.5 line. If, at the next examination, the visual acuity has reduced to 6/9 owing to active pathology, this will be missed because the examiner would not realize there had been any change in visual acuity.

Sheridan–Gardiner test This test is designed to assess visual acuity in young or intellectually impaired patients. It consists of five booklets containing single-letter optotypes on each page. Three booklets assess visual acuity from 6/60 to 6/18, 6/18 to 6/6, and 6/6 to 6/3 respectively, with three letters at each visual acuity level to prevent familiarization of the letters from confounding the results. The fourth booklet has one letter at each visual acuity level and can be used to assess visual acuity from 6/60 to 6/6.

The test is designed to be used at 6 m, but may be used at 3 m by halving the visual acuity values, or at 6 m with use of a mirror.

There is also a booklet for measuring reduced Snellen visual acuity and near visual acuity in N notation.

Sonksen–Silver card

This test is suitable from about 3.5 years of age and presents letters in linear format. It includes letters that are spaced at intervals equal to the width of one letter, in order to introduce contour interaction in the horizontal direction.

LogMAR acuity charts

This chart was designed to overcome many of the shortcomings of the Snellen chart. There are several different versions of this chart but all adhere to the original principles described by Bailey and Lovie in 1976, and all work in the same way (Fig. 2.2). Internal (back-lit) and external illuminated versions are available. The advantages of the chart are:

- There are five letters on each line.
- Spacing between each letter and each row is related to the width and height of the letters respectively.
- Each row is a scaled-down version of the row above.
- The task remains the same as the patient reads down the chart, and therefore results obtained at different viewing distances can easily be equated.
- The progression of letter sizes is uniform, increasing in a constant ratio of 1.26 (0.1 log unit steps).
- The result is noted in terms of a logMAR score (log minimum angle of resolution); 6/6 is equivalent to a logMAR of zero ($\log_{10}$ of $1 = 0$), and 6/60 is equivalent to 1 ($\log_{10}$ of $10 = 1$).
- Smaller letters have a negative logMAR score because $\log_{10}$ of any number less than 1 is negative.
- Large letters have a positive score.
- As letter size changes in units of 0.1 log units per row, each letter has been assigned a score of 0.02 (five letters on each line).
- The final logMAR score takes into account every letter that has been read correctly, no matter what line it was read from.
- However, as with the Snellen chart, contour interaction is not equal across each line and the letters at each end are easier to identify.

LogMAR acuity test (Keeler crowded–uncrowded cards)

This chart comprises three sets of cards and a key card for letter-matching in patients who are unable to name letters. Two sets are designed to measure crowded linear visual acuity and are identical apart from differing arrangement of letters, while the third set consists of cards with two widely spaced uncrowded letters on each card (Fig. 2.3).

The test is usually performed at a distance of 3 m in a well illuminated room. In the sets designed to measure crowded linear visual

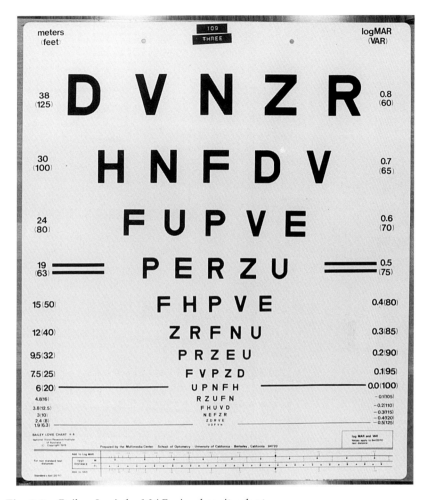

Fig. 2.2   *Bailey–Lovie logMAR visual acuity chart.*

acuity there are four letters on each line (chosen from six: XVOHUY) of approximately equal legibility, with all letters being symmetrical about the vertical midline.

Other features include the following:

- The visual demand on each line is constant.
- Each line on the chart represents a change of 0.1 log units in acuity level, and each letter has a value of 0.025 log units.
- At 3 m, the chart and the examiner are more likely to be within the sphere of interest of the child. Measured visual acuity ranges from 6/38 to 6/3 at 3 m.
- The initial visual acuity level can be determined using the screening cards (cards 1–3 in each of the crowded tests). The last successful response on the screening cards is used to determine the starting point for the measurement of linear visual acuity. Using this technique an estimation of the patient's visual acuity can be made and

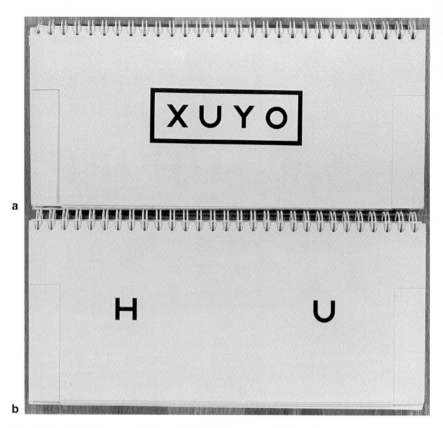

Fig. 2.3   *(a) Keeler crowded card. (b) Keeler uncrowded card.*

then refined quickly, as it is not necessary for all the test cards to be used.
- The test is highly portable and of low cost, but good external illumination is required.
- Visual acuity can be recorded in metric Snellen, logMAR and modified logMAR (reciprocal of logMAR) notation.

Kay pictures

This chart is designed for young children who are unfamiliar with letters (2–5 years of age) and may also be useful when assessing intellectually impaired people of any age.

The test consists of easily recognizable shapes, such as a house, with one shape on each page. A 'recognition booklet' is provided to help determine how the child interprets each shape (Fig. 2.4). For example, the house shape may be interpreted as home or school. This information can then be used when the test is conducted.

There are 3- and 6-m versions; both use metric Snellen notation.

A disadvantage of the test is that it uses single optotypes and therefore has no crowding effects. A logMAR version is also available.

LH distance acuity symbols

The Lea Hyvärinen (LH) chart is suitable for children aged 18 months and above, and is available in both single and crowded formats. It has

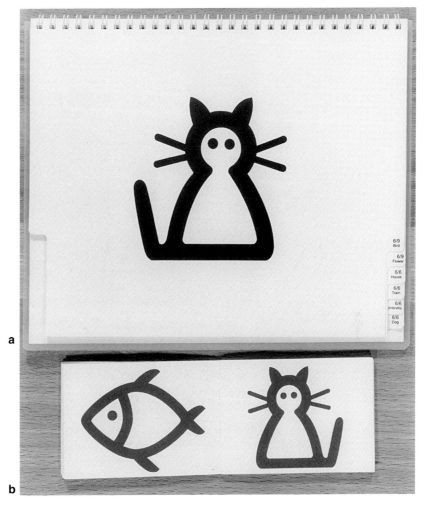

Fig. 2.4   *(a) Kay pictures with (b) recognition booklet.*

the following features:

- Symbols are uniform in detail, line width and overall size, providing a more standardized visual acuity task.
- The test is based on four symbols – house, heart (or apple), circle and square – which blur equally; i.e. all symbols are equally sensitive to blur and equally difficult to distinguish. This means that, when blurred, all the symbols appear to the observer to be circles.
- The patient can still believe themselves to be answering 'correctly', while the examiner can easily detect the visual acuity threshold without revealing to the child that they have failed to recognize the symbol.
- The symbols are easy to name, sign or point to on a key card, or with the help of separate three-dimensional symbols that match the chart symbols in appearance.
- Versions with internal (back light) or external illumination are available.

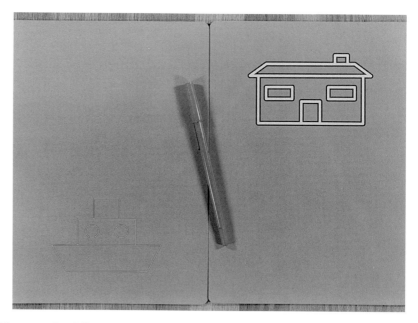

Fig. 2.5   *Cardiff acuity card.*

Cardiff acuity cards

These cards are designed to measure visual acuity in children aged 1–3 years, but can be used in older children and adults with intellectual impairment. Use of the cards includes the following features:

- The targets are described as vanishing optotypes and consist of a white band boarded by two black bands, each half the width of the white band and all on a neutral grey background (Fig. 2.5).
- The average illuminance of the target is equal to that of the grey background. If the target lies beyond the subject's visual acuity limit, it merges with the grey background and becomes invisible.
- The targets are all of the same size, but the black and white bands decrease in width. Visual acuity is recorded as the narrowest white band for which the target is visible.
- The test uses the principle of preferential looking: an infant will choose to look towards a target rather than towards a plain stimulus.
- The cards are held with a vertical orientation in front of the child at either 50 cm or 1 m, depending on where the child's attention can be obtained (a working distance of 1 m is recommended whenever possible).
- It is important that the examiner is unaware of the location of the target (bottom or top) and should present each card without looking at the front where the optotypes are printed.
- The examiner judges in which direction the child is looking (up or down).
- Three cards are included at each visual acuity level, although only two are usually presented. Once one card has been presented, neither child nor examiner can predict the position of the target on the next card to be presented.

- The vertical orientation of the card allows easier discrimination in cases of nystagmus.
- If the direction of gaze of the child and the position of the target are the same, another card with finer lines is presented.
- For any given target width, if the examiner estimates the target position incorrectly, or is unable to make a judgement from the child's responses, the target is assumed to be beyond the child's visual acuity limit.
- The endpoint is taken as the visual acuity level at which at least two out of three cards are scored correctly.
- At 1 m, the visual acuity range measured is from 6/60 to 6/6, and at 50 cm the range is from 6/120 to 6/12.

Keeler acuity cards

This is a preferential-looking grating test. Grating and preferential looking tests tend to give a higher acuity than a letter test simply because the observer is required only to resolve the target and not to identify it:

- The patterns utilized are square-wave gratings (Fig. 2.6) described in terms of their spatial frequency – the number of black and white pairs in each degree of visual angle.
- The higher the spatial frequency, the finer the grating.
- The grating is placed in a circle with a white border; to prevent edge effects from confounding the results, there is also an empty circle on the grey side of the card.

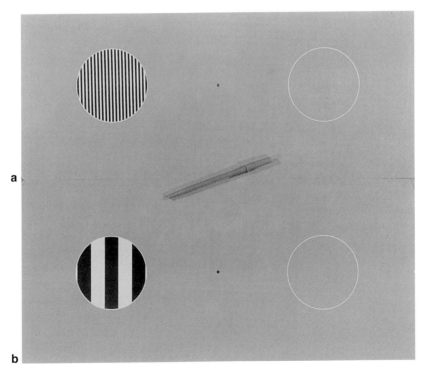

Fig. 2.6 *Two Keeler acuity cards, a) high spatial frequency, b) low spatial frequency.*

- The stimulus and blank have equal average luminance.
- When the stimulus is beyond the resolution limit the viewer, the card will appear to have two grey patches of equal luminance within the white circles; under these circumstances the infant will show no looking preference.
- The design ensures that the visual acuity estimate is based on the ability to detect and resolve the grating rather than a preference for one shade of grey over another.
- Gratings of increased spatial frequency are presented to an infant and their looking responses are recorded.
- The highest spatial frequency (finest grating) that elicits an appropriate looking response is used to estimate visual acuity.

Near reading acuity and visual acuity

Faculty of Ophthalmologists near reading acuity card

This is a chart used in many optometric practices. As it consists of words in context and not individual letters, it does not assess near visual acuity but near reading acuity.

It uses N notation: the number following the N corresponds to point size, with one point being equal to 1/72 of an inch (Fig. 2.7). The range is from N5 to N48, and there are various versions with various passages of text. Readers should remember that N5 is approximately equivalent to 6/9 at 25 cm, and therefore patients are rarely tested to threshold.

Use of the chart includes the following:

- Pathology can be missed. For example, if a patient has N3 reading acuity at 35 cm, this will be recorded as N5 at 35 cm. If the patient later presents with subtle retinal disease and the reading acuity at 35 cm has decreased to N5, the practitioner will be unaware of this clinically significant change.
- The chart has also been criticized for not simulating a real-world task, because of the high contrast between the letters and the background.
- Reading acuity should be recorded monocularly and binocularly, and any asymmetry noted. Most versions also have music, classified advertisements and technical drawings, so that some functional testing is possible.
- It is common practice to assess the near reading acuity with the use of additional localized lighting, such as that provided by an Anglepoise lamp. A reduction in reading speed when the lamp is switched off can be used to demonstrate the importance of localized lighting to older people.
- A requirement of many patients is to be able to read newspaper-sized print; N8 is approximately equivalent to column newspaper print in size, but probably not in contrast. It is important to ask the individual to read out loud, because an interocular change in reading speed or accuracy may indicate macular dysfunction.
- The preferred reading distance should be measured to the nearest 1 cm and recorded with the N number that corresponds to the smallest size of print read at this distance.
- An N number without reading distance is a measurement of size and not of reading acuity. This applies to all reading acuity and near visual acuity charts.

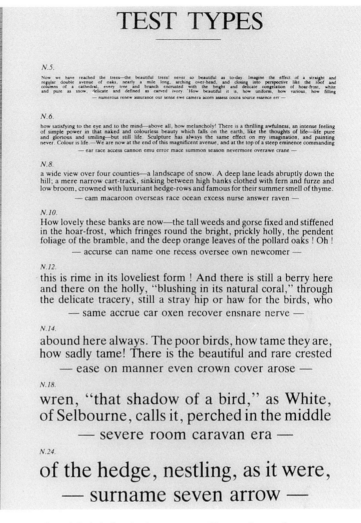

Fig. 2.7 *Faculty of Ophthalmologists near reading acuity card.*

Maclure reading chart and bar reading book

This can be used to measure reading acuity in young children. The reading material has been chosen by a specialist in the teaching of reading and is based on the reading ability expected for different age groups of children. Each age has been given a grade, numbered from 1 to 7, so that even if a child's reading ability is not equal to the average age, the grade number can be used to give an indication of reading acuity. The Maclure chart includes the following:

- Within each grade, specimens of printing in sizes N5 to N48 have been used (Fig. 2.8).
- The chart attempts to relate text to age. The structure of the text changes in terms of word and line length and of difficulty.
- Each book also contains a 6-m distance chart with lower-case or 'school script' letters, a standard 6-m Snellen chart and reduced Snellen and 'school script' distance charts that must be used at 35 cm.

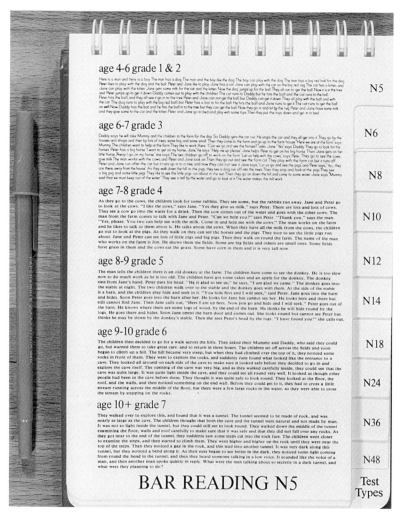

Fig. 2.8 *Maclure book.*

LogMAR near visual acuity letter chart

This is similar in design to the logMAR distance acuity test, with five letters on each of 17 lines. The chart has all the advantages associated with a logMAR design (see p. 8) and also the one disadvantage: less crowding at the end of each line of letters. As the chart is comprised of individual letters, it does measure near visual acuity and not reading acuity.

Near visual acuity can be recorded in terms of M units (1M corresponds to the resolution of a 5° target at 1 m and roughly equates to newspaper-sized print), decimal and reduced Snellen (metric and imperial) notation. For the logMAR visual acuity values printed on the card to be valid, the working distance has to be 40 cm.

The chart is usually printed on both sides with a different series of letters to avoid the learning effects when right and left and binocular visual acuity are measured.

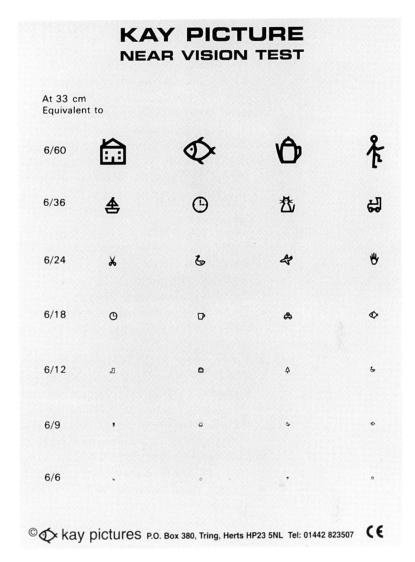

Fig. 2.9   *Kay picture near vision test.*

Kay picture near vision test

This consists of a single card with seven rows, and four symbols on each row (Fig. 2.9). The symbols are identical to those used in the 3- and 6-m and logMAR versions. Although described as a near vision test, it is really a way of measuring equivalent Snellen visual acuity (range from 6/60 to 6/6) at 33 cm. This test may be of use in situations where it is difficult to gain the cooperation of a young child when using charts with much greater testing distances.

LH symbols near acuity chart

This is similar in design to the LH distance acuity chart, and uses the same house, heart (or apple), circle and square symbols.

Institute of Optometry near test card

This chart builds on recent research on visual acuity assessment yet retains a fairly familiar appearance. It is easy to use for clinicians who are accustomed to conventional designs, and includes the following features:

- It is produced as an A5-sized laminated card.
- It consists of a column of isolated words and allows a rapid estimate of visual acuity. The words are simple and can be read by young or poor readers, and are arranged in random order with a logarithmic progression in size.
- The chart uses point size units (e.g. N6).
- A conversion table is included, enabling point size to be converted to logMAR, decimal, imperial Snellen and metric Snellen notation.

Practical near acuity chart (PNAC)

- This is a single card with a print size range from N80 to N5, with a regular decreasing progression of 0.1 logMAR, with high-contrast lower-case Times Roman font, and N, M (1M is equivalent to N8) and logMAR notation (figures printed on card are valid only when the testing distance is 25 cm).
- There are 13 rows with three related words per row. Each row has one three-letter, one four-letter and one five-letter word, totalling 12 letters.
- When using logMAR notation, each three- and four-letter word should be scored at 0.03 logMAR, and each five-letter word at 0.04 logMAR (adding to 0.10 logMAR units for each line).
- When using N notation, the patient can be asked to hold the card at their habitual reading distance; this then needs to be noted along with the N value for the smallest words read.
- The word reading threshold is reached when fewer than two words on a row are read correctly.
- Several word sequences for the chart are available to reduce learning effects with repetition.
- The words used have been chosen to be easily recognizable by people with the educational ability of an average 9 year old.
- The reverse side of the card contains commonly used print sizes, so fluency and reading speed can be tested once near visual acuity threshold has been established.

Bailey–Love near word reading card

- This is a single card with a print size range from N80 to N2, with a regular decreasing progression of 0.1 logMAR, with high-contrast lower-case Times Roman font, and N, M and logMAR notation (figures printed on card are valid only when testing distance is 40 cm).
- There are 17 rows of unrelated words: the first three rows have two words, the next three rows have three words, and the remaining rows have six words (Fig. 2.10). Therefore, the task varies according to which part of the card is used.
- The threshold is reached when more than 50% of the words on a row are read incorrectly.

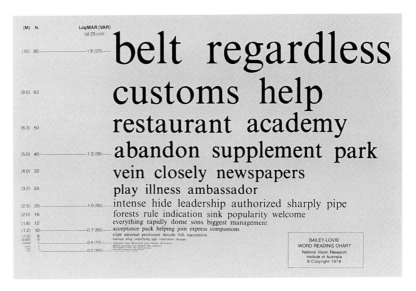

Fig. 2.10   *Bailey–Lovie near word acuity card.*

- Several word sequences for the chart are available to reduce learning effects with repetition.
- Clinical experience suggests that use of this card can be slow with children and those with poor language reading or cognitive skills.

3

The cover test

Introduction

The cover test can be defined as an objective dissociation test to elicit the presence of a heterotropia or heterophoria. It relies on the observation of the behaviour of the eyes whilst fixation is maintained and each eye is covered and uncovered in turn. It is important to adapt the method and choice of target to the patient's age, refractive status and type of deviation found. For example, an accommodative stimulus should be used for a young person, especially when the deviation is thought to have an accommodative element, but this is less important for a presbyope, when a light stimulus will suffice. Figure 3.1 shows the basic equipment needed to carry out the cover test.

Prerequisites

Refractive status

- For children and some adults, the cover test should be performed with and without any refractive correction in situ (see Patients 1 and 8 on the CD video clips).
- For pre-presbyopic adults, the cover test should be performed with and without any refractive correction in situ (for most myopes use the refractive correction for a 6-m testing distance).
- For presbyopic adults who require refractive correction, the cover test should be performed with the refractive correction in situ.

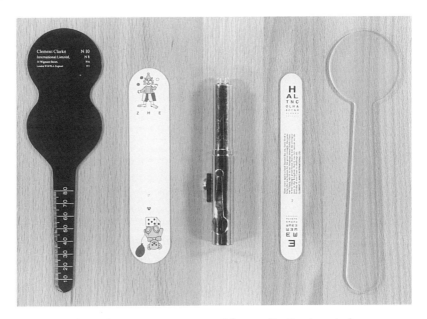

Fig. 3.1 *Basic equipment; opaque cover stick, near fixation targets for young children, pen torch, near fixation targets for older patients, translucent cover stick.*

● For all patients, if prisms are incorporated into the refractive correction then the cover test should be performed with and without refractive correction in situ, using appropriately sized targets.

Compensatory head posture

The cover test should be performed with and without the compensatory head posture (CHP) to assess the effect of the CHP on the control of the deviation (see Patient 13 on the CD).

Primary position

The patient should fixate the target at eye level to ensure that all the extraocular muscles are equally in tone. It is our experience that novices assess near cover test movements in depression and not primary position of gaze.

Diplopia

In comprehending verbal patients, ask how many targets are seen. A single image in the presence of an obvious heterotropia implies suppression.

Fixation targets

The choice depends on the level of visual acuity of each eye and on the intellect of the patient.

Testing distance

6 m

● If visual acuity is less than 6/18 in either eye, a spotlight target is most appropriate.
● A target further away than 6 m may be used when the deviation is greater at 6 m than at 33 cm.

33-cm testing distance using a spotlight target

● Observation of corneal reflections – a large-angle kappa may displace the corneal reflexes nasally but this displacement is symmetrical.
● Presence of central, eccentric or wandering fixation.
● Reveals the presence or absence of accommodative component to a deviation when compared with the results using an accommodative stimulus.

33-cm testing distance using an accommodative target

● Testing with an accommodative target is appropriate for pre-presbyopic patients.
● Use of a detailed target will ensure that accommodation is being exerted. Any change in the size of deviation compared with the size observed with a spotlight target should be noted.

Clinical procedure

Cover–uncover test

The aim is to elicit the presence or absence of a heterotropia. One eye is covered and the uncovered eye is assessed for any movement to refixate (see demonstration on CD-ROM).

Information obtained from the cover–uncover test

Type of deviation (Figs 3.2–3.5)

● Direction (horizontal, vertical, torsional or a combination)
● Unilateral or alternating
● Constant or intermittent
● Effect of refractive correction
● Effect of accommodation
● Effect of CHP.

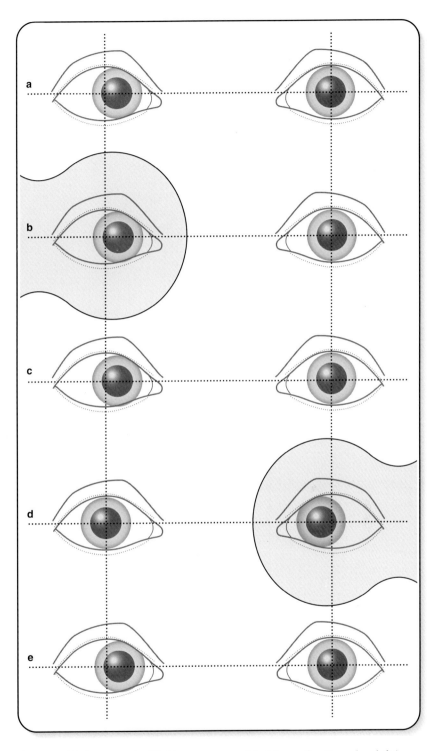

Fig. 3.2 *Right esotropia. Right eye moves out to take up fixation when left is covered (d). Can be observed using unilateral cover–uncover test.*

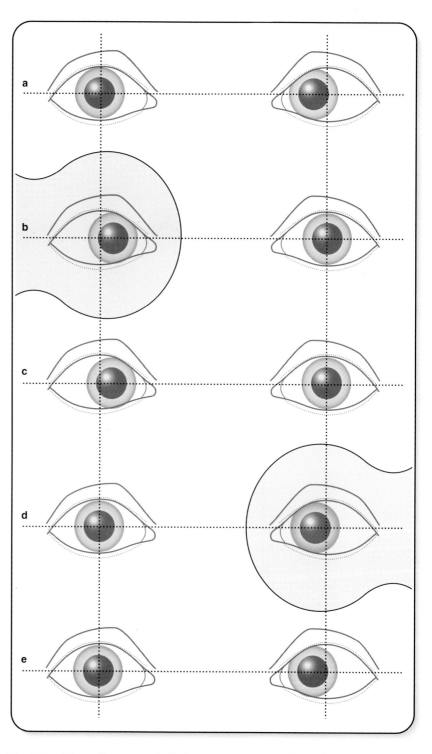

Fig. 3.3 *Alternating esotropia. Left eye moves out to take up fixation when right is covered (b). Right eye moves out to take up fixation when left is covered (d). Can be observed using unilateral cover–uncover test.*

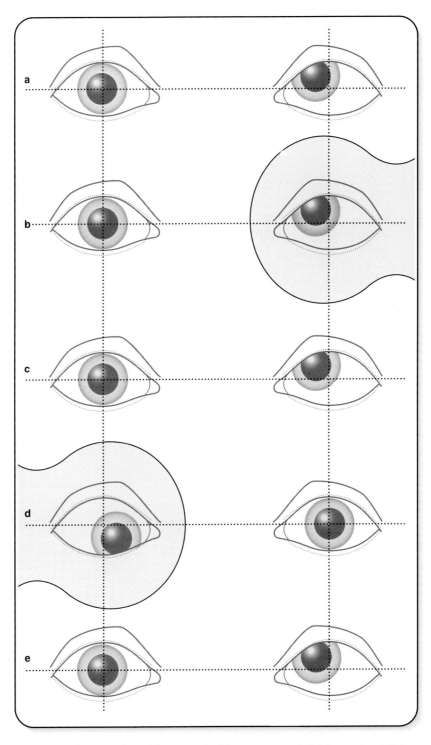

Fig. 3.4 *Left esotropia and hypertropia. No movement of right eye when left is covered (b). Left eye moves down and out when right is covered (d). Can be observed using unilateral cover–uncover test.*

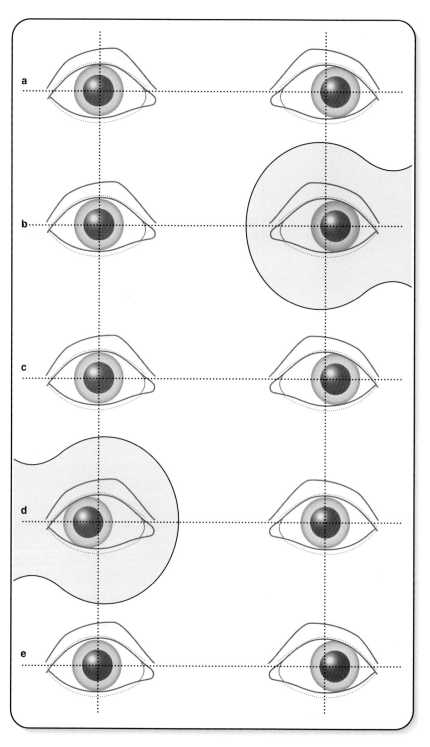

Fig. 3.5   *Left exotropia. No movement of right eye when left is covered (b). Left eye moves inwards when right is covered (d). Can be observed using unilateral cover–uncover test.*

Size of deviation

- Hirschberg's reflection test (Fig. 3.6): each millimetre of displacement from the centre of the cornea equates to approximately 15 prism dioptres (Δ) of deviation (see p. 47 for Method).
- Comitant or incomitant.

Fixation

- Central (foveal) or near central (parafoveal)
- Eccentric
- Wandering.

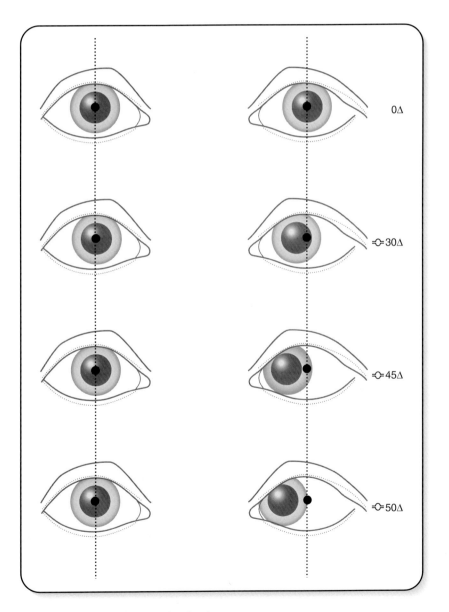

Fig. 3.6 *Hirschberg's corneal reflections.*

Visual acuity

- Speed of uncovered eye to take up fixation can be used to indicate level of visual acuity in the deviating eye (e.g. slow uptake implies poor visual acuity).
- Alternating deviations indicate equal visual acuity.
- Objection to occlusion of one eye may indicate poor visual acuity in the uncovered eye.

Associated phenomena

- Manifest and latent nystagmus – manifest nystagmus is apparent before the occluder is introduced, whereas latent nystagmus is elicited when one eye is occluded.
- Dissociated vertical divergence – the eye behind the occluder will elevate and extort, associated with latent nystagmus (Fig. 3.7).

Alternate cover test

The aim is to elicit the presence or absence of a heterophoria. One or other eye is covered throughout the test, i.e. complete dissociation is achieved and the patient is never binocular during the test.

- Movement of the eye behind the occluder as it is moved to the other eye should be noted.
- To ensure maximum dissociation, each eye should be covered three or four times in turn for about 2 seconds each time.
- The rate of recovery of the covered eye when the occluder is removed should be noted.
- The alternate cover test is fully dissociative and reveals the total deviation but it should not be used to differentiate between heterophoria and heterotropia (see demonstration video on the CD-ROM).

Information obtained from the alternate cover test

Type of deviation (Figs 3.8–3.11)

- Effect of refractive correction
- Effect of accommodation
- Effect of CHP.

Size of deviation

- Excursion to take up fixation on recovery
- Comitant and incomitant
- Incomitancy can indicate either anisometropia or a paralytic strabismus.

Recovery movement

- Rate of recovery – the speed at which this occurs relates to the quality of fusion and the control of the deviation
- Recovery – full to bifoveal fixation; partial to small-angle heterotropia (usually a microtropia)
- Rate of recovery – a difference in speed of excursion between either eye can indicate a difference in visual acuity.

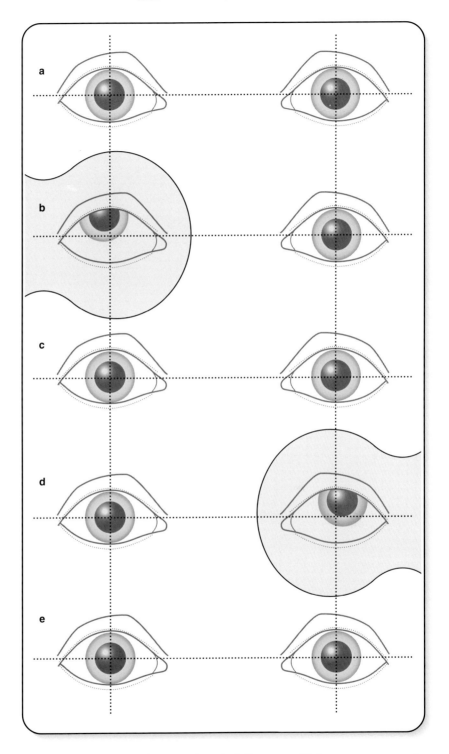

Fig. 3.7 *Asymmetrical dissociated vertical divergence. Right eye moves up and out when covered (b), and recovers on cover removal (c). Left eye also moves up and out when covered (d) and recovers on cover removal. Can be observed using unilateral cover–uncover test. Note, in this particular example there is no deviation until one or other eye is covered.*

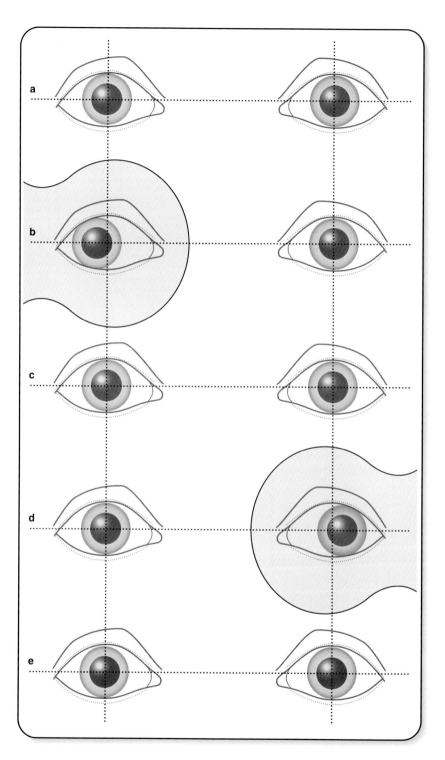

Fig. 3.8   *Exophoria. Eye under cover moves out (b, d). Inwards recovery movement when cover is removed. Best observed using alternate cover–uncover test.*

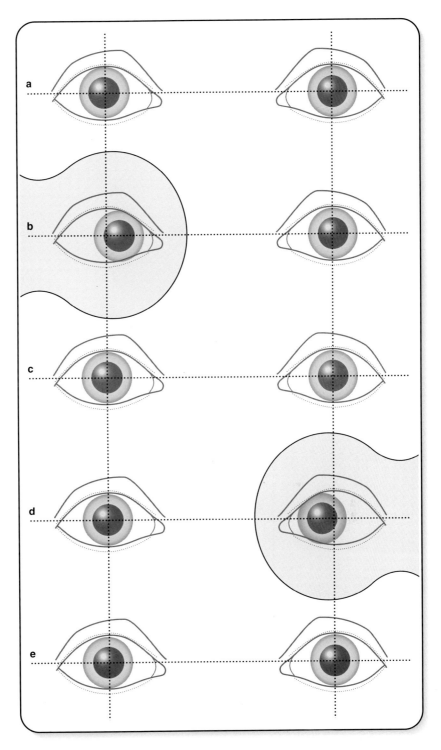

Fig. 3.9 *Esophoria. Eye under cover moves in (b, d). Outwards recovery movement to take up fixation when cover is removed. Best observed using alternate cover–uncover test.*

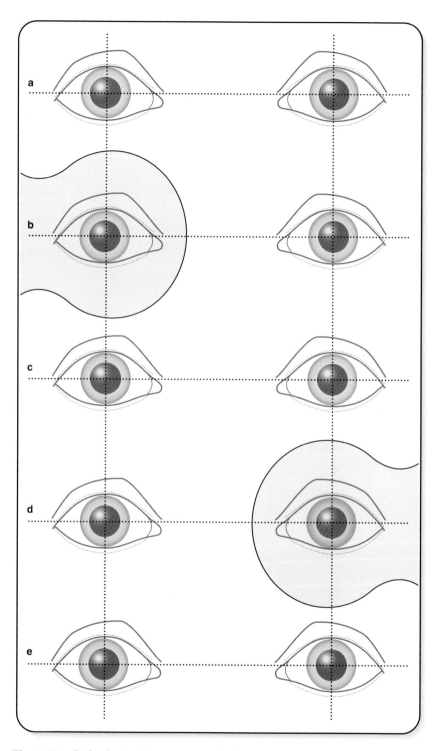

Fig. 3.10 *Orthophoria. No movement of either eye on covering with either unilateral cover–uncover or alternating cover test.*

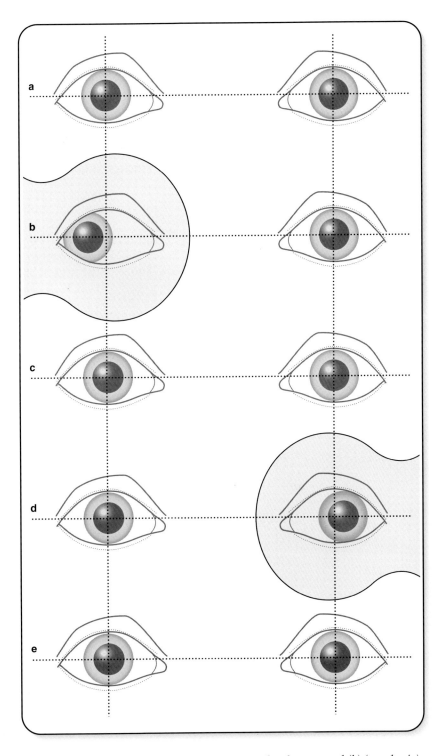

Fig. 3.11 *Anisophoria. Right eye moves outwards when covered (b) (exophoria). Left eye moves outwards when covered (d) but to a lesser extent than the right eye (b). Best observed using alternate cover–uncover test.*

Associated phenomena
- Latent nystagmus.
- Diplopia prior to delayed recovery implies poor control of the deviation.
- Dissociation induces decompensation of the deviation.

Use of the cover test with other tests

Ocular movements

The alternate cover test can be conducted in the nine primary positions of gaze during objective oculomotility to determine the presence of underacting or overacting muscle(s) (see Ch. 8).

Binocular visual acuity

- Used to elicit the maximum visual acuity achieved while maintaining BSV.
- Intermittently, a rapid cover–uncover test is performed while the patient reads down the vision chart, to determine whether decompensation occurs. This is indicated by a reduction in reading speed and accuracy.

4

Assessment of refractive error

Introduction

Detailed description of objective and subjective refraction is beyond the scope of this book and is well covered in other texts. Here we will concentrate on techniques that are useful when standard distance fixation refraction is not possible. It is imperative to obtain an accurate measurement of any refractive error, because BV anomalies are often associated with significant refractive error. When working with young children, the practitioner must be adaptable in terms of working distance, should use hand-held spheres rather than trial frames, and must be quick for conclusive results to be obtained.

Cycloplegic refraction

This is useful for babies and young children when there is strabismus, suspected refractive error or reduced vision:

- The drug of choice is cyclopentolate, preferably in non-preserved single-dose form. For children younger than 12 months of age, 0.5% cyclopentolate should be administered (as their small liver and kidneys mean reduced ability to metabolize drugs, increasing the chance of an adverse drug reaction with a greater dosage) and 1% for children older than this.
- Most young children are nervous about the application of eye-drops and there may be resistance to instillation.
- One way of overcoming this is to persuade the child to close their eyes and place a single drop in the inner canthus of each eye. As the child opens their eyes and blinks, enough of the drug will enter the eye to produce cycloplegia and mydriasis.
- Refraction should then take place 30 minutes later, in reduced illumination, with the child fixating the retinoscope at 50 cm.
- Loose trial lenses quickly placed in front of each eye to neutralize the retinoscopy reflex allow the refractive error to be determined.
- The working distance of 50 cm (equivalent to –2.00DS) can then be subtracted from this value.
- No tonus allowance should be made in the presence of strabismus, and maximum plus and minimum minus should be prescribed.
- If there is no strabismus, a further 0.50 to 1.00DS (depending on the size of the refractive error found) should be subtracted to give the final result.

Near fixation retinoscopy (Mohindra technique)

If there is suspected allergy to cyclopentolate or the child is not cooperative for the instillation of drops, the Mohindra technique can be used as an alternative:

- Room lights need to be extinguished completely and the child encouraged to fix the retinoscope light (this produces very little accommodative stimulus in a dark room). One eye should be occluded; this is easily achieved with the hand that is holding the trial lens.

- Research has shown that for 2-year-old children, reducing the final result by −1.25DS produces a result that is close to that obtained by cycloplegic refraction.
- For children aged less than 2 years, the result should be reduced by −1.00DS.

Brückner test

The purpose of this test is to assess the symmetry of binocular fixation by comparing the brightness of the red reflex in each of the two eyes. A difference in brightness may be caused by anisometropia, strabismus, anisocoria, media opacities or posterior pole abnormalities, however it is not possible to determine the nature of amount of refractive error using this technique.

- Shine a direct ophthalmoscope toward the patient's eyes from a distance of 80–100 cm using a large round patch of light to illuminate both pupils simultaneously, and instruct the patient to look at the centre of the light.
- Looking through the peep-hole of the direct ophthalmoscope, the examiner should dial in the lens that gives a clear view of the patient's pupils.
- While observing Hirschberg's reflexes against the red reflex in the pupil, the brightness of each red reflex can be compared. If the two reflexes are equally bright, there is binocular fixation.
- If the reflexes are not equally bright, the darker red reflex indicates the normal eye, and the brighter, lighter, or whiter reflex indicates the abnormal eye.
- Note how this contrasts with the use of a retinoscope, when the reflex of the affected eye is usually darker.

5

Tests of accommodative function

Introduction

Clinical tests of accommodative dysfunction can be grouped into four categories: amplitude of accommodation, accommodative facility, tests that directly or indirectly assess lag of accommodation, and relative accommodation.

Amplitude of accommodation

- This is a measure of the maximum amount of accommodation that an individual can exert and is usually measured using a Royal Air Force (RAF) rule with the smallest text readable (Fig. 5.1).
- Accommodative testing should be conducted monocularly and binocularly, and repeated at least three times for each situation in order to test for fatigue.
- Young children should be advised to read the smallest line that they can resolve to themselves. The presence of saccadic eye movements would indicate that the child is attending to the task; accommodation will be engaged and accurate results obtained.

Accommodative facility

- This is a measure of the speed of accommodative change.
- The dioptric accommodative stimulus is alternated between two different levels and the subject reports when a letter target (Fig. 5.2) is seen clearly after each alternation in accommodative stimulus.

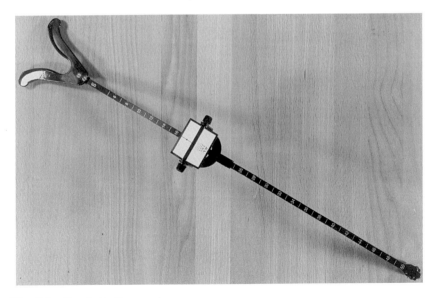

Fig. 5.1 *Royal Air Force rule.*

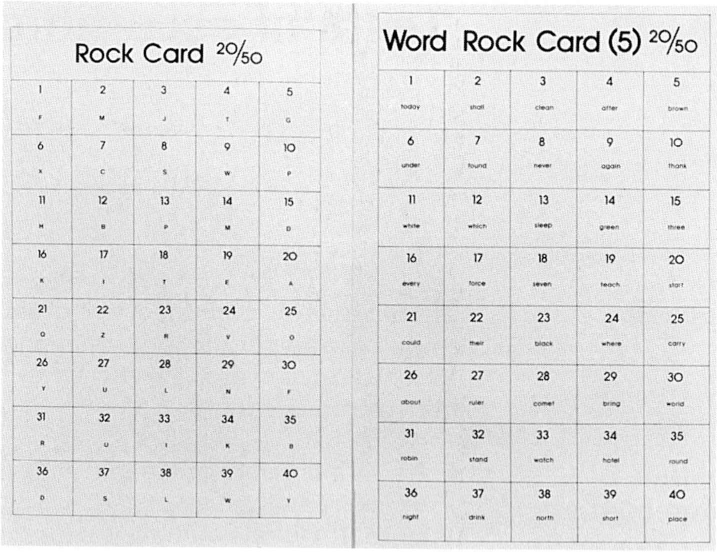

Rock Card ²⁰⁄₅₀

1	2	3	4	5
f	M	J	T	Q
6	7	8	9	10
K	C	S	W	P
11	12	13	14	15
H	B	P	M	D
16	17	18	19	20
K	I	T	E	A
21	22	23	24	25
Q	Z	R	V	O
26	27	28	29	30
Y	U	L	N	F
31	32	33	34	35
R	U	I	K	B
36	37	38	39	40
D	S	L	W	Y

Word Rock Card (5) ²⁰⁄₅₀

1	2	3	4	5
today	shall	clean	after	brown
6	7	8	9	10
under	found	never	again	thank
11	12	13	14	15
white	which	sleep	green	three
16	17	18	19	20
every	force	seven	teach	start
21	22	23	24	25
could	their	black	where	carry
26	27	28	29	30
about	ruler	comet	bring	world
31	32	33	34	35
robin	stand	watch	hotel	round
36	37	38	39	40
night	drink	north	short	place

Fig. 5.2 *Hart charts for accommodative facility testing using 'lens rock'.*

- The examiner counts the number of cycles completed in 1 minute (one cycle being the change from one stimulus level to the other and back again).
- The accommodative stimulus can be varied either by lens power changes or by viewing distance changes.
- The first is referred to as 'lens rock' and the second as 'distance rock', indicating that the accommodative stimulus is 'rocked' back and forth.
- The standard method of testing accommodative facility is a lens rock procedure using a pair of +2.00DS lenses on one side of a flipper bar and −2.00DS lenses on the other side (Fig. 5.3).
- The test starts with the +2.00DS lenses over the subject's refractive correction. A test distance of 40 cm is usually used with the reduced Snellen letters at a 6/6 to 6/12 acuity demand (Hart charts).
- However, this type of target has no suppression control, and for children younger than 6 years of age it is more appropriate to use the OXO target on the near Mallett unit. With the polarizing filters in place, the vertical fixation disparity bars can be used to check for suppression.
- During binocular 'lens rock' testing, adjustments in fusional vergence must occur to compensate for the changes in accommodative vergence. Therefore, subjects may pass the monocular lens rock but fail the binocular lens rock facility if a vergence disorder is present.
- Cut-offs for test failure used by many clinicians, with +2.00DS/ −2.00DS flippers and a 40-cm viewing distance for children and adults up to 30 years of age, are less than 11 cycles per minute for monocular testing and less than 8 cycles per minute for binocular testing.

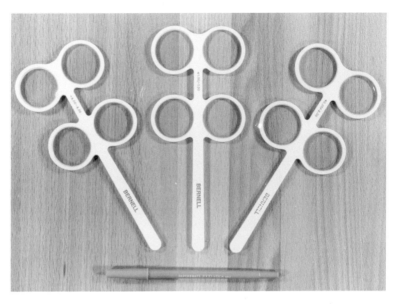

Fig. 5.3   Accommodative facility: flipper bars for lens rock method.

Lag of accommodation

- During accommodation for near-point viewing, the retina is usually conjugate with a point slightly behind the object of regard. For near-point targets, accommodative response is usually slightly less than the accommodative stimulus.
- The amount by which the dioptric accommodative response is less than the dioptric accommodative stimulus is the lag of accommodation.
- This category of accommodation tests can be further divided into: (1) tests that measure the lag of accommodation and (2) tests in which lens power is changed to alter accommodative stimulus to the point at which dioptric accommodative stimulus and dioptric accommodative response are equal.
- A test card with an aperture in the centre is used so that the examiner can observe the retinoscopic reflex close to the subject's visual axis through the aperture.

Monocular estimate method

This is an example of a test that measures lag of accommodation. In the monocular estimate method (MEM), the amount of the lag of accommodation is estimated by judging the width, speed and brightness of the retinoscope reflex:

- The test card (Fig. 5.4) and the retinoscope are placed at the same distance from the subject's spectacle plane, usually 40 cm.
- With the retinoscope in the plane mirror mode, 'with' motion indicates a lag of accommodation and an 'against' motion indicates a lead of accommodation. Neutrality indicates that the accommodative stimulus and accommodative response are equal.

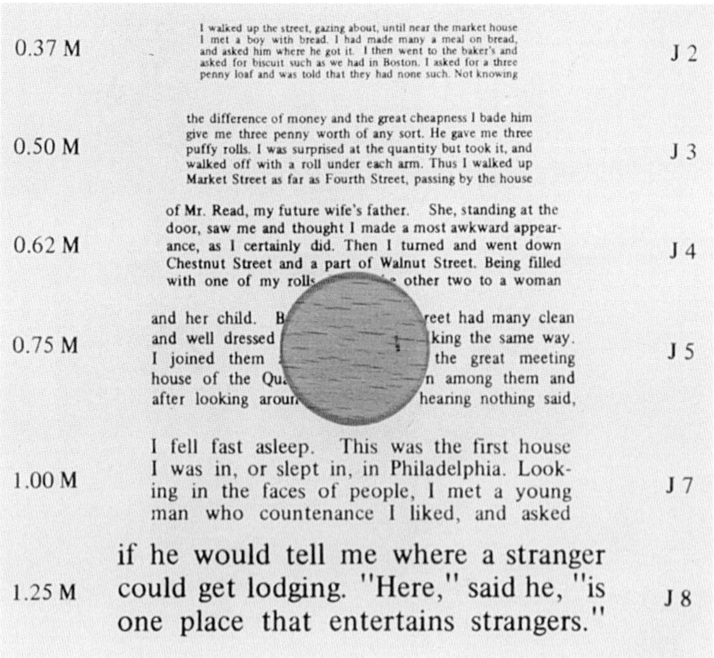

| 0.37 M | I walked up the street, gazing about, until near the market house I met a boy with bread. I had made many a meal on bread, and asked him where he got it. I then went to the baker's and asked for biscuit such as we had in Boston. I asked for a three penny loaf and was told that they had none such. Not knowing | J 2 |

the difference of money and the great cheapness I bade him give me three penny worth of any sort. He gave me three puffy rolls. I was surprised at the quantity but took it, and walked off with a roll under each arm. Thus I walked up Market Street as far as Fourth Street, passing by the house — 0.50 M — J 3

of Mr. Read, my future wife's father. She, standing at the door, saw me and thought I made a most awkward appear-ance, as I certainly did. Then I turned and went down Chestnut Street and a part of Walnut Street. Being filled with one of my rolls...the other two to a woman — 0.62 M — J 4

and her child. B...reet had many clean and well dressed...king the same way. I joined them...the great meeting house of the Qua...n among them and after looking aroun...hearing nothing said, — 0.75 M — J 5

I fell fast asleep. This was the first house I was in, or slept in, in Philadelphia. Look-ing in the faces of people, I met a young man who countenance I liked, and asked — 1.00 M — J 7

if he would tell me where a stranger could get lodging. "Here," said he, "is one place that entertains strangers." — 1.25 M — J 8

Fig. 5.4 *Monocular estimate method (MEM) test card.*

- The examiner's estimate of the amount of plus power that would be required to neutralize the 'with' motion is the estimate of the lag of accommodation.
- The estimate of the lag can be confirmed by briefly placing a plus lens equal in power to the estimated lag over one eye and quickly checking to see whether neutrality is observed.
- The lens should be in place for only half a second or less, so that a change in accommodative response is not induced.
- School-aged children are reported to have a mean lag of 0.34DS.
- Most non-presbyopic subjects have lags of 0 to 0.75DS with MEM retinoscopy.

Low neutral dynamic retinoscopy

This is a test that makes use of lenses to measure accommodation. Low neutral dynamic retinoscopy yields the lens power with which the diop-tric accommodative stimulus and dioptric accommodative response are equal:

- The retinoscope and the test card are maintained at the same dis-tance from the subject, usually 40 cm from the spectacle plane.
- Testing is started with the subject's distance refractive correction in place.
- If a lag is observed, plus lenses are added in 0.25DS steps until a neutral retinoscopic reflex is observed.
- The lens power added for neutrality is recorded. If, for example, the test result is +0.75DS with a 40-cm distance, the accommodative stim-ulus is 0.75DS less than the 2.50DS for the test distance, or 1.75DS.

- As the neutral was observed at that point, the accommodative response is also 1.75DS.

Relative accommodation

Values are elicited using plus-to-blur (or negative relative accommodation; NRA) and minus-to-blur (or positive relative accommodation; PRA) tests. These are usually conducted with the use of a photopter, as measurements are difficult with a trial frame:

- The subject is instructed to view a near target, usually at 40 cm, through the distance refractive correction.
- Positive lenses are added until the test target becomes blurred. These are removed and then negative lenses are added until the target again becomes blurred.
- This is also an indirect assessment of the vergence system, as the vergence demand remains constant while the accommodative demand varies.

6

Practical application of prisms

Introduction

Prisms can be used for both diagnostic and therapeutic purposes. In this chapter only their diagnostic uses will be discussed.

Objective measurement of the angle of deviation

Prism cover test

This is an objective dissociative method of measuring the total angle of deviation using horizontal and vertical prisms. Torsional deviations cannot be measured.

- Angles of deviation should be measured at 6 m and 33 cm in the primary position of gaze.
- The test may also be used to measure deviations at other distances and fields of gaze, depending upon findings from the history, cover test and ocular motility assessment.
- Results from the cover test and ocular motility will provide information on the approximate size and components of the deviation, the preferred eye for fixation, and whether the deviation is comitant or incomitant.

Equipment
- Horizontal and vertical prism bars and loose square prisms (Fig. 6.1).
- Detailed fixation targets, selected appropriately for the age of the patient and level of visual acuity of each eye.
- Occluder (for younger patients, the palm of the examiner's hand may be more suitable).

Prerequisites
- Cooperative patient.

Method
- The patient is required to fixate a target at 6 m. A prism strength approximating the size of the deviation should then be placed in front of the deviating eye in heterotropia or either eye in heterophoria, and, if the deviation is incomitant, with the apex in the direction of the deviation.
- An alternate cover test should be performed gradually increasing the prism strength until the movement of the eye is reversed. The size of the deviation is recorded as the prism value just before reversal.
- The procedure should be routinely repeated for 33 cm and, when indicated, in other fields of gaze (maintain the fixation target in the primary position while the patient's head is moved to place the eyes

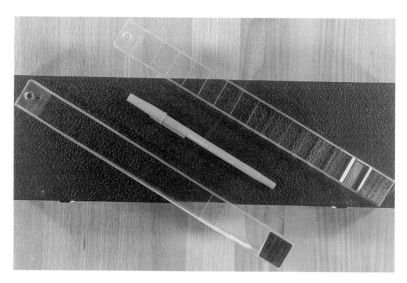

Fig. 6.1   *Prism bars.*

in the required position), fixation distances, and when fixing with each eye in the case of heterotropia.

Precautions

It is essential to:

● prevent fusion and elicit the total deviation – for maximum dissociation allow sufficient time (2 seconds) for the patient to fixate the target accurately, followed by a quick movement of the occluder to the other eye;
● maintain and control accommodation by using a detailed fixation target appropriate for the patient's age.

Simultaneous prism cover test

This is a modification of the prism cover test and is used to measure the heterotropic component of a deviation that has heterotropic and heterophoric components, for instance in some cases of microtropia.

Method

Results of the cover test reveal the coexistence of a heterotropic and heterophoric deviation, when assessment of the size of the heterotropia enables more accurate classification of the type of deviation.

● The prism is placed in front of the deviating eye and a cover–uncover test is performed only on the fixing eye.
● Prism and cover are removed and the test repeated with larger prisms.
● The deviation is therefore measured using minimum dissociation until the point of reversal. The size of the manifest component is recorded as the prism value just before reversal.
● See Hirschberg's method also (p. 47).

Prism and reflection test   This is an objective method of determining the total objective angle of a deviation. It is useful in the testing of children, patients who are unable to cooperate with the prism cover test, and when bifoveal fixation is absent.

Method

- The patient fixates a spotlight at 33 cm in the primary position.
- A prism bar (or loose prism) is placed in front of the deviating eye with the prism apex in the direction of the deviation.
- The prism strength is increased until the corneal reflection of the deviating eye is positioned in the same relative position as that in the fixating eye.
- This method is appropriate only for measurement at near.

Krimsky test

This is a variation of the prism and reflection test.

Method

- The patient fixates a spotlight at 33 cm in the primary position.
- Prisms are placed in front of the fixating eye.
- Prism strength is increased until the reflex is centred in the pupil of the deviating eye.
- This method is appropriate only for measurement at near.

Subjective measurement of the angle of deviation

This is a subjective dissociative test designed to measure the size of a heterophoric deviation at 33 cm.

Maddox wing

Equipment

- The instrument is hand-held and consists of two slit apertures and trial lens holders, one for each eye, and a septum with a plate fixed to the end bearing measurement scales.
- The left eye sees a horizontal and vertical measurement scale calibrated in degrees. The right eye sees two arrows: one vertical to indicate the horizontal deviation and one horizontal to measure the vertical deviation.
- To assess the presence of torsion, a white scale of 2° divisions and a red horizontal arrow are situated on the right-hand side of the plate.

Method

- The instrument should be held in a slightly depressed position with any near refraction correction in situ.
- The patient is asked to indicate the position of the vertical arrow on the horizontal scale to record the horizontal deviation, and the position of the horizontal arrow on the vertical scale to measure the vertical deviation.
- Torsion is present if the horizontal arrow is not parallel with the horizontal measurement scale on the plate. The patient is asked to move the arrow until it is perceived as being parallel.

Maddox rod

This is a subjective method for measuring heterophoric horizontal, vertical and torsional deviations (Fig. 6.2). The eyes are dissociated by presenting a spotlight to one eye and a coloured line image to the other eye.

Prerequisites

- Normal retinal correspondence
- Cooperative patient
- All other light sources should be turned off.

Equipment

- Maddox rod (in trial lens or hand-held form, usually red in colour). The rod consists of a series of parallel high-power plano-convex cylinders that convert a point source of light into a line image at 90° to the cylinder axes.
- This test can be conducted at 6 m and 33 cm.

Method

The test is performed fixing with either eye at 6 m and 33 cm, and with the patient's refractive correction in situ.

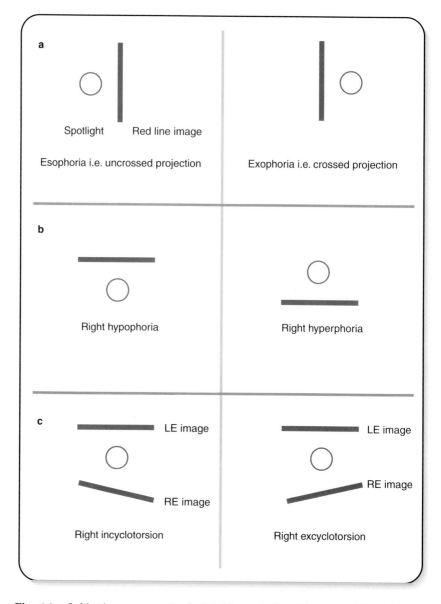

Fig. 6.2 *Subjective responses to the Maddox rod, placed in front of the right eye. (a) Horizontal heterophoria. (b) Vertical heterophoria. (c) Maddox double rod for cyclotorsion.*

Horizontal deviations

- The Maddox rod is placed in front of one eye with the cylinders placed horizontally.
- The patient fixates a spotlight and is asked to report on which side of the spotlight the vertical red line is positioned.
- Horizontal prisms are placed and adjusted in front of one eye until the patient reports that the line passes through the spotlight.

Vertical deviations

- The cylinders are placed vertically, producing a horizontal red line.
- Measurement is made using vertical prisms.

Torsional deviations

- Two Maddox rods in a trial frame are placed in front of each eye with the cylinder axes positioned exactly vertical, producing parallelhorizontal line images.
- To facilitate recognition of any tilt, a low-powered vertical prism can be placed in one side of the trial frame.
- Measurement is made by rotating the rod until the patient reports that the two lines are exactly parallel.
- Torsion is recorded in degrees according to how much the rod in front of the non-fixing eye was rotated.

Estimation of the angle of deviation

This is a test for estimating the objective angle of a heterotropia at 33 cm.

Hirschberg's method

Method

- The patient observes a spotlight at 33 cm in the primary position.
- The examiner notes the position of the corneal reflection in the fixating eye and compares it with the reflection in the deviating eye (see Fig. 3.6).
- The angle of deviation can be estimated on the correlation that each 1 mm of displacement, relative to the corneal reflection in the fixating eye, is equal to 12–15 prism dioptres (Δ) (see Patient 10 on the CD).

Fusional vergence

Prisms can also be used to measure fusional vergence (Fig. 6.3).

Components of fusional vergence

- Sensory fusion – the ability to appreciate two similar images, one formed on each retina, and interpret them as a single image.
- Motor fusion – the maintenance of sensory fusion during vergence movements.

Implications

- If sensory and motor fusion are present, the prognosis is good.
- Conservative and surgical management is directed to obtaining a functional outcome. Sensory fusion alone may be insufficient to maintain a stable eye position.
- If fusion is absent, conservative treatment is contraindicated and any operation would be for cosmetic reasons.
- The strength of motor fusion is represented by the fusion amplitude, comprising horizontal, vertical and cyclovergence.
- The fusion range correlates to the quality of binocular single vision.

Horizontal fusion amplitude

Positive reserves

- Assess the near point of convergence first, noting which eye (if any) diverges on failure of convergence to determine the dominant eye and whether the patient appreciates diplopia.

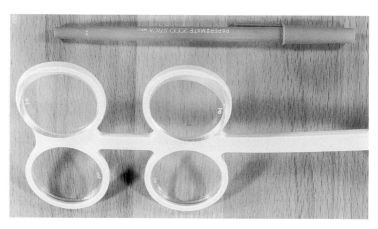

Fig. 6.3   *Vergence facility flipper prisms.*

- The prism bar should be placed base out in front of the dominant eye to facilitate observation of the non-dominant eye (Fig. 6.4). If the patient recognizes diplopia, measurement can be made objectively and subjectively. Initially use prism with a base direction that opposes the heterophoria, e.g. for an exophoria use base-out first and then base-in. If suppression is present on failure of convergence, measurement is made objectively and the examiner records when the non-dominant eye ceases to make a fusional movement.

Method
- The patient fixates a detailed target, to stimulate accommodation, at 33 cm in the primary position.
- The strength of prism is slowly increased and the patient is asked to report the point at which the target blurs (blur point) and whether and when diplopia is recognized (break point).
- The prism strength is slowly reduced until fusion is restored (recovery point).
- The amplitude is recorded as the highest powered prism that can be overcome by fusion.
- The blur, break and recovery components of the fusion range can thereby be documented and compared on subsequent assessments.
- Repeat for 6 m.

Negative reserves

Precaution
- Use a spotlight target at 33 cm and 6 m to facilitate observation of the break point and to relax accommodation.

Method

Use base-in prisms and then as for positive reserves.

Vertical fusion amplitude

The vertical amplitude comprises supravergence (prism base down) and infravergence (prism base up). Measurement is useful in assessing the ability to compensate for a vertical deviation and whether it is of recent onset or long-standing.

Method
- The patient fixates a detailed target at 33 cm in the primary position.

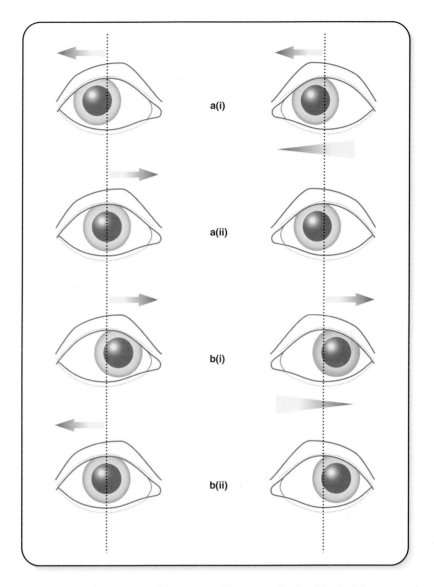

Fig. 6.4 *Prism fusion range. (a) Base out: (i) image is displaced in the left eye, away from fovea to temporal macula; both eyes make a conjugate movement to the right according to Hering's law of equal innervation; (ii) to overcome the induced disparity, the right eye makes a refixation disjugate movement to the left to regain binocular single vision (BSV). (b) Base in: (i) image is displaced in the left eye, away from fovea to nasal macula; both eyes make a conjugate movement to the left, according to Hering's law of equal innervation; (ii) to overcome the induced disparity, the right eye makes a refixation disjugate movement to the right to regain BSV.*

- Vertical prism strength is slowly increased until the patient recognizes diplopia.
- Repeat for 6 m.

Normal fusion amplitude	*Distance*	*Convergence*	*Divergence*	*Vertical*
	33 cm	35–40Δ BO	10–12Δ BI	3Δ BU to 3Δ BD
	6 m	15–20Δ BO	5–7Δ BI	3Δ BU to 3Δ BD

where BO = base out, BI = base in, BU = base up, and BD = base down. These values apply to the prism bar and will be different when measured using an instrument such as the photopter.

Vergence facility

Vergence facility can be assessed with prism flippers (see Fig. 6.3). It is defined as the number of cycles per minute that a stimulus can be fused through alternating base-in and base-out prism, and it attempts to capture the ability of the fusional vergence system to respond rapidly and accurately to changing vergence demands over time, measuring stamina and sustaining ability. The last-mentioned refers to the ability to maintain vergence at a particular level (rather than to rapidly alter the level) for a sustained period of time and is assessed by holding the prism flipper in front of the eyes until the subject experiences ocular discomfort.

Various combinations of base-in and base-out prisms have been described in the literature, including 4 base-in/16 base-out, 5Δ base-in/15Δ base-out and 8Δ base-in/8Δ base-out. We currently use 6Δ base-in/18Δ base-out. With 4Δ base-in/16Δ base-out flippers one study showed that 5-year-olds had a mean of 7.6 cycles/min and 12-year-olds had a mean of 13.0 cycles/min. With the 5Δ base-in/15Δ base-out and 8Δ base-in/8Δ base-out flippers mean values were similar for the two tests, ranging from 11.3 to 14.1 cycles/min. Some clinicians put less emphasis on the number of cycles per minute and more on the quality of vergence movements, i.e. any discomfort, grimacing or tendency to pull away from the flippers. The ease with which the subject overcame the prisms can be noted.

20/15/10-Dioptre base-out prism test

The main use of this test is to determine the presence of sensory and/or motor fusion, and therefore to differentiate between a pseudo-heterotropia and a true deviation. It is particularly useful as a screening test in children.

Principle

A base-out prism (preferably in loose form) held before one eye will shift the image of the fixation object on to temporal retina, inducing crossed diplopia. The patient needs to make a positive fusional movement to regain binocular single vision. The prism strength has to be large enough to produce a noticeable eye movement but not so high powered that fusion of the images becomes difficult. The 10-dioptre prism is more suitable for infants, progressing up to 20 dioptres for school children when vergences are fully developed.

Four-dioptre prism test

This is an objective test to detect the presence or absence of bifoveal binocular single vision. It is indicated in cases of heterotropia and anisometropia where unequal visual acuity exists, to determine whether there is a central suppression scotoma (Fig. 6.5). The test is used with the prism base out for suspected microesotropia and with the base in for microexotropia (where all the movements described below will be in the opposite direction).

Equipment

- Four-dioptre loose prism or horizontal prism bar
- 6-m fixation target.

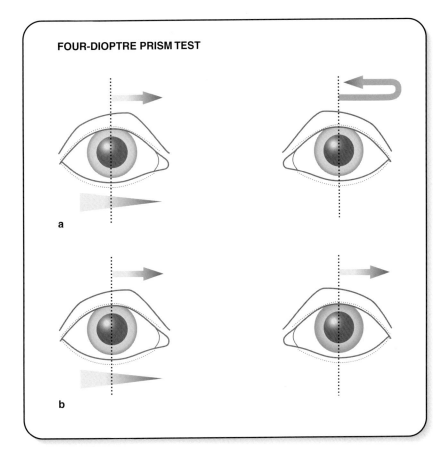

Fig. 6.5 *Four-dioptre prism test. (a) Fusion response in bifoveal binocular single vision. (b) Central suppression scotoma response in left microtropia with identity.*

Method
- Observation of results is more apparent at a fixation distance of 6 m using a detailed target.
- The prism is placed base out in front of the eye with the best visual acuity, and the examiner notes the movement of the other eye.
- Repeat for the other eye.

Results
- Bifoveal BSV is confirmed if the suspect eye makes a rapid inward movement to regain foveal fixation (Fig. 6.5a).
- An eye with a central suppression scotoma will remain outward (owing to Hering's law of equal innervation) with no corrective movement (Fig. 6.5b). On placing the base-out prism in front of the suspect eye, there will be no movement as the image falls within the area of the central scotoma.

AC/A ratio

The AC/A ratio determines the amount of accommodative convergence induced in response to 1 dioptre of accommodation. The normal ratio is 2–4 : 1, i.e. 2–4 dioptres of convergence is produced from each dioptre of accommodation. Unless there is surgical intervention, the ratio is maintained until the onset of presbyopia. If the ratio is higher or lower than normal, overconvergence or underconvergence may produce a heterotropia.

Indications for measurement

The size of the ratio is important in certain cases and is used to determine whether management should take a conservative or surgical course. Measurement is indicated in:

- all cases in which there is a significant difference between the size of the distance and near deviations
- intermittent esotropia of the convergence excess type
- intermittent distance exotropia to differentiate between true and simulated types.

Methods

There are several methods of measurement, but only the gradient method will be discussed here, as it is easily conducted in clinical practice. The gradient method can be used with concave lenses at 6 m for convergence excess deviations, or convex lenses at 33 cm for divergence excess deviations.

Concave lenses

- With any refractive correction in situ in a trial frame, the deviation is measured with the prism cover test at 6 m using a detailed fixation target.
- With –3.00DS lenses in a trial frame, the distance prism cover test should be repeated using the same target, provided it can still be seen clearly.
- If sufficient exertion of accommodation is not possible, the ratio should be calculated using either –2.00DS or –1.00DS.

Calculation of ratio

$$AC/A = \frac{(PCT \text{ value in active state} - PCT \text{ value in non-active state})}{\text{Strength of lens used}}$$

where PCT = prism cover test, BO = base out, and BI = base in.

For example, for convergence excess esotropia:

PCT with –3.00DS = 25Δ BO
PCT without –3.00DS = 4Δ BO
AC/A ratio = (+25 – (+4))/3 = 7 : 1 (i.e. a high ratio).

Convex lenses

The method is the same as for concave lenses, but the fixation target should be at 33 cm and convex lenses used.

If the patient cannot relax the accommodation by 3 dioptres, then either +2.00DS or +1.00DS can be used. For example, for distance exotropia:

PCT without +3.00DS = 10Δ BI
PCT with +3.00DS = 35Δ BI to the nearest whole number
AC/A ratio = (–10 – (–35))/3 = 8 : 1 (i.e. a high ratio).

7

Tests to determine binocularity

Suppression

Two types of suppression exist:

- *Physiological suppression* – present in normal BSV to prevent aware-ness of physiological diplopia and retinal rivalry.
- *Pathological suppression* – develops to overcome symptoms:
  — binocular diplopia – occurs in heterotropia when the image of an object stimulates a non-corresponding point in the deviating eye. The diplopia is overcome by peripheral suppression.
  — confusion (rarely a symptom) – occurs in a heterotropia when the fovea of the fixating eye receives the image of the object but the fovea of the deviating eye receives the image of an object in the peripheral field that lies on its visual axis. Both foveal images are superimposed and projected to the same point. Confusion is overcome by central suppression.
  — incompatible images – occurs in BSV when the same object stim-ulates each fovea but the retinal images are different in size and/or shape and prevent central fusion. Peripheral fusion maintains binocular single vision but central suppression occurs in the more ametropic eye.

Area of suppression

In heterotropia, suppression involves two areas: the fovea of the devi-ating eye and the point that corresponds with the fovea of the non-deviating eye. In esotropia, these two types of suppression areas merge to form an elliptical scotoma with its long axis horizontal (also known as Lang's D-shaped scotoma). The size of the scotoma corre-lates with the size of the deviation. In exotropia, the area suppressed is not thought to be as definitive, ranging from a suppression scotoma similar to that found in esotropia to suppression involving the whole of the temporal retina.

Investigation of suppression area

Using prisms

Method

- Either a detailed target or a spotlight (viewed through red and green goggles) is fixated by the patient at 33 cm.
- Prisms are placed in front of the deviating eye and gradually increased in strength until the patient appreciates diplopia.
- The area can be mapped out by changing the prism base direction and repeating this procedure.

Binocular status test

In some types of heterophoria, the BVS can be considered to be under 'stress'. In order to reduce the stress, the fovea of one eye is sup-pressed while the rest of the retina functions normally. A simple way of testing for foveal suppression is to use the 'binocular status' test on the Mallett near vision unit.

Principle

When the polarizing visor is in place, the central letters on this mini-Snellen chart are seen binocularly and therefore provide a foveal lock, whereas other letters, which are cross-polarized, are seen monocularly. The left eye sees letters on the right of this chart and the right eye sees those on the left.

Method

- The test should be performed at 33 cm with any required spectacle correction and the polarizing visor in place with good ambient illumination.
- If the patient does not read some of the letters it is necessary to determine whether this is due to foveal suppression or to reduced monocular near acuity.
- The simplest way to determine this is to occlude the other eye; if the missing letters can now be read, they were originally missed because of foveal suppression (a binocular phenomenon).
- If the letters are still missing when the patient is tested monocularly, there is a near acuity problem.
- It is possible to determine the angular subtense of the suppressed area because the letters are graded in minutes of arc, from 20 to 5 minutes.
- Note that the type of suppression described here is associated with heterophoria and not heterotropia.

Density or depth of suppression

Suppression associated with heterotropia is densest when central and becomes progressively less dense as the scotoma extends into the periphery.

Measurement

The Sbiza (Bagolini filter) bar consists of a series of filters increasing in colour density from very pale pink to very dark red, numbered from 1 to 17. The bar gradually reduces the illumination of the spotlight image in the fixing eye to induce awareness of the image in the deviating eye, and therefore diplopia. It is used to assess the depth of suppression and to monitor the likelihood of intractable diplopia as an outcome of occlusion therapy in cases approaching visual maturation.

Method

- The patient is asked to fixate a spotlight at 33 cm in the primary position of gaze.
- The Sbiza bar is then introduced in front of the fixing eye at filter 1.
- The density of the filter should gradually be increased until the patient reports one white and one pink/red spotlight. Sometimes the filter bar may act as an occluder: the red spot changes to a white spot and the patient will then not report diplopia.
- The filter number at which diplopia occurs indicates the depth of suppression.
- A neutral density filter bar can also be used.

Diagnostic tests for suppression

Tests are designed to assess recognition of diplopia. The method required to elicit diplopia can be used to indicate the depth of suppression.

Peripheral suppression

Method
- Septum – if suppression is superficial, diplopia may be recognized by holding a card perpendicular to the patient's nose.

For more dense suppression:

- Red filter in front of suppressing eye observing a spotlight.
- Red and green filters in front of either eye.
- Worth's four lights test (see section on retinal correspondence).

Central suppression

Methods
- Four-dioptre prism test (see section on uses of prisms).

Mallett unit

As well as being used to detect fixation disparity, the Mallett unit (Fig. 7.1) can be used to detect suppression associated with heterotropia.

Method
- Fixation disparity tests are best performed when the refractive error, including any presbyopic addition, is in the trial frame.
- The Mallett unit is held at the patient's normal reading or working distance, which may be exactly measured using the retractable tape measure incorporated in the housing of the unit.
- The patient should first be asked to read a few words from the text surrounding one the OXO targets.
- The patient should then be directed to look at the X of the OXO, and to be aware – but not directly look at – the green markers. Without the Polaroid visor in place the markers should appear to be centrally aligned with the X; this gives the patient a reference point of how the markers should be positioned.
- The visor can now be placed in the trial frame and the patient asked whether two green markers are still visible – one above and one below the X. If only one line is seen, there is dense central suppression in the eye that corresponds to the missing marker.
- If there is no suppression, both strips will be seen and the patient is asked whether the top strip is exactly above the bottom strip. If this is the case, there is no retinal slip and any heterophoria that is present is compensated (Fig. 7.2).
- If the top strip (which is seen by the left eye) is to the right of the bottom strip, an exodisparity is present. The patient is then asked whether only one line has moved from the cross, demonstrating a slip in only one eye, or whether both have moved, indicating a slip in both eyes.
- If the slip is in the other direction, the patient has an uncompensated esophoria.
- The patient is then directed to the OXO with horizontal green markers, again fixating the cross, and asked whether the two green strips are exactly level, indicating orthophoria or compensated hyperphoria, or whether one line is slightly higher than the other.

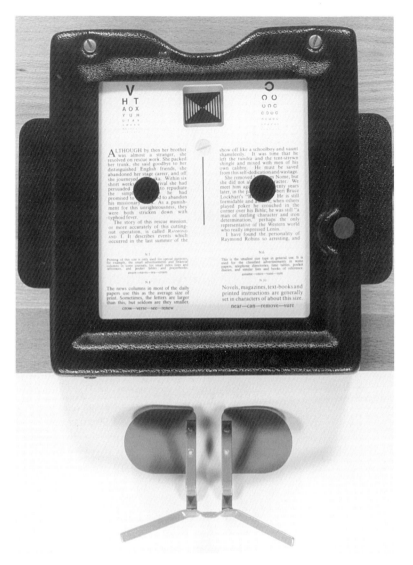

Fig. 7.1   *A version of the near Mallett unit.*

- As the left strip is seen with the right eye, the left strip will appear higher than the right in uncompensated left hyperphoria, and vice versa in right hyperphoria.
- Again, it should be noted whether the slip is in the right or left eye, or is bilateral.
- Cyclophoria is thought to be prevalent in near vision, but seldom causes problems. Cases of uncompensated cyclophoria can be detected by the sloping of one or both green strips.

Key point

The slip will subtend only 5–15 minutes of arc and, although this is easily seen by all but the most unobservant patient, some patients may expect the strips to separate widely and regard a small separation as insignificant and not worthy of mention. Any displacement is important – however small it may appear to the patient.

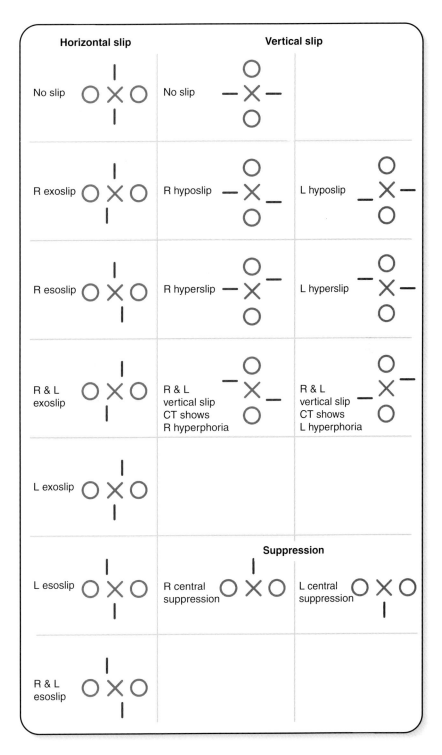

Fig. 7.2 *Mallett unit analysis. R, right; L, left. Horizontal slip = top marker seen by left eye, bottom marker seen by right eye. Vertical slip = left marker seen by left eye, right marker seen by right eye.*

- Slip can be eliminated by means of prisms or spheres, starting with low values (±0.25DS or 0.5Δ) and gradually increasing the strength until the slip disappears; between changes of prism or sphere, the patient should read two or three lines of print surrounding the target to stabilize the accommodative response.
- Sometimes only 1Δ is required to eliminate the fixation disparity; this should not be ignored and clinical experience has shown us that a lateral prism as small as 1Δ or a vertical prism of 0.5Δ eliminates the symptoms.

Binocular instability

This condition may occur with an uncompensated heterophoria. In these cases there is usually some variation in the amount of prism or sphere required to eliminate the horizontal slip on the Mallett unit and the markers tend to oscillate across the neutral point; alternating suppression often results from this binocular instability. It is occasionally deep enough for one of the green strips to fade or even disappear. Small positive and then negative spheres should be introduced if movement is reported to stabilize the markers, followed by base-in or base-out prism if the spheres fail.

Determination of AC/A ratio (see Ch. 6)

The target used for detecting lateral fixation disparity on the Mallett unit provides a convenient method for investigation of this relationship.

Principle

If the patient exhibits a lateral slip, the minimum prism is found that will eliminate it; with the prisms removed, the minimum binocular spheres are then found that achieve the same result.

Method

- If 4Δ (divided between each eye) is required or –2.00DS were needed to remove the slip, the relationship (prism/lens ratio) would be 2Δ/1DS.
- If the patient does not show a fixation disparity, this can first be induced with prisms and then repeated with spheres, with base-in prisms and minus spheres or with base-out prisms and plus spheres. The minimum power of prism and spheres that causes a slip to develop will give the required relationship.
- The normal relationship is thought to be of the order of 2–4Δ/1DS.

Detection of the dominant eye at near

The non-dominant eye is the one that readily relinquishes binocular fixation or foveal vision when the binocular vision system is stressed. The stress may be inherent as, for example, in decompensated heterophoria, or it may be induced artificially using equal prisms placed in front of both eyes.

  If the patient exhibits a uniocular slip, the eye that retains fixation is the dominant eye; where no slip is apparent it may be induced, with prisms divided equally between the eyes.

  Where the slip, whether induced with prisms or present because of an uncompensated heterophoria, is present in both eyes, it can be safely assumed for clinical purposes that no marked ocular dominance is present.

Prism adaptation

For binocular vision disorders, it is often wise to investigate whether the patient does adapt to prism before prescribing it.

Method

- The proposed prism should be 'trial framed' and worn by the patient for five minutes.
- During this trial period the patient should read or perform a visual task likely to be done with the prescribed prescription.
- If, after this period, the patient's alternate cover test magnitude or fixation disparity through the prism is larger than that which was predicted to be measured through this prism power, prism adaptation is likely to be occurring and the prism will probably not benefit the patient in the long term.

Stereopsis and stereoacuity

Stereopsis can be described as binocular visual depth perception based on retinal rivalry; it is assessed qualitatively. Stereoacuity can be described as a measurement of the stereoscopic threshold derived from the minimum disparity that results in the appreciation of depth. It can be measured quantitatively in seconds of arc.

- *Local stereopsis* – This is detected with stereograms that have individual elements such as lines, edges or contours, such as the Wirt circles found in the Titmus stereo test (see below for details of this test). However, these features are often visible monocularly as well as binocularly, although monocular cues are not as obvious when the polarizing filters are in place.
- *Global stereopsis* – This is detected using random dot stereograms such as the Lang I and II, and the TNO test. The visual system pools together information from the entire stereogram to create a global perception of depth and form. This is a more complex visual task than the detection of local stereopsis.

Qualitative test for stereopsis

Lang's two-pencil test

- The examiner holds a pencil vertically in front of the patient.
- The patient is asked to place another pencil directly on top of the examiner's pencil.
- The test is performed with both eyes open and then with the 'weaker' eye covered.
- The responses are compared.

Results

- In patients with heterotropia, a more accurate response with both eyes open indicates anomalous BSV.
- In patients with no apparent heterotropia, a more accurate response with both eyes open denotes BSV. Further tests would be necessary to confirm whether it is bifoveal.
- In patients whose responses are similar, this implies monocularity.
- This test is useful to differentiate between a pseudo-deviation and a true deviation in young children.

Quantitative tests for stereoacuity

Tests based on random dots or shapes

These tests have target areas in which dots or other shapes are identical but are displaced horizontally in relation to one another to create the disparity. All other areas are filled with random dots or shapes that do not correspond with either eye.

TNO test

- Based on random dots printed as red and green anaglyphs (Fig. 7.3).
- Viewed through red and green glasses at a test distance of 40 cm.
- Consists of seven plates: three gross stereo plates, one suppression plate and three graded plates containing segmented circles with disparities ranging from 480 to 15 seconds of arc.
- No monocular cues.
- Suitable for children (aged about 4 years and upwards) and adults.

Lang stereotest

- Combines the use of random dots and panography. The targets are seen alternately by each eye, and are then fused to create the disparity.
- The Lang I test consists of three targets – a cat, a star and a car – with disparities ranging from 1200 to 550 seconds of arc.
- The Lang II test consists of four targets – a star (which acts as a control and is visible to patients who are monocular), a car, an elephant and a moon – with disparity reaching 200 seconds of arc (Fig. 7.4).
- To avoid monocular cues, the cards should be presented parallel to the plane of the patient's face and the patient encouraged to sit still.
- These tests are most suitable for screening purposes.

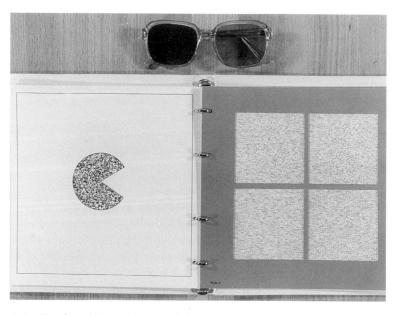

Fig. 7.3 *Random dot TNO test graded plate.*

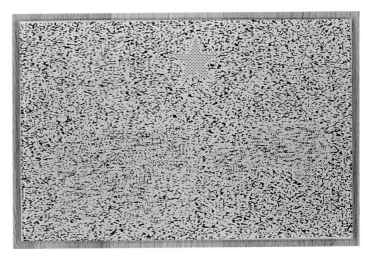

Fig. 7.4 *Lang II test with the monocular star target clearly visible.*

Frisby stereotest

- Based on random triangular shapes without displacement, the test consists of three plastic plates of different thickness: 6, 3 and 1 mm.
- Each plate has four squares of shapes (Fig. 7.5): one square contains a circle of shapes which is printed on the back surface of the plate, giving a three-dimensional effect.
- Disparity varies with the thickness of the plate and with the viewing distance, ranging from 600 to 15 seconds of arc.
- The disparity can be altered from crossed to uncrossed by reversing the plate; by rotating the plates, the position of the circle can be changed.
- The plates need to be held parallel to the plane of the patient's face to avoid the use of parallax to reveal the circle.
- Can be used with young children through to adults. In our experience, objective testing with infants as young as 6 months is achievable.

Tests using polarization

These tests are based on the principle of polarized stereography, consisting of two polarized images at right angles to each other. When viewed through polarized spectacles, the image seen by one eye is polarized at 90° to that seen by the other eye.

Titmus stereotest

- Consists of two plates, held at a test distance of 40 cm (Fig. 7.6).
- One plate has an image of a house-fly. Stereoacuity of approximately 3000 seconds of arc is demonstrated if the wings of the fly are perceived in three dimensions. Care should be taken in that this target may frighten some children.
- The second plate consists of nine sets of four circles (Wirt circles). One circle from each set is displaced to create disparity, ranging from 800 to 40 seconds of arc.

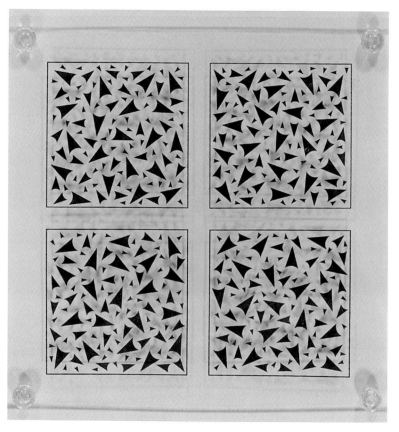

Fig. 7.5 *Frisby test.*

- Beneath the circles are three rows of animals. Disparity of between 400 and 100 seconds of arc can be demonstrated if one of the animals in each row is seen in three dimensions.
- Monocular cues present on the circles (not so obvious when viewed monocularly with the filters in place) are particularly evident with the first three sets. Therefore, results are to be interpreted cautiously.

Randot stereotest
- Similar in principle to the Titmus stereotest; consists of two plates held at a test distance of 40 cm (Fig. 7.7).
- One plate contains six random dot shapes, giving a range of disparity of from 500 to 250 seconds of arc.
- The second plate consists of circles, measuring from 400 to 20 seconds of arc, and three rows of animals with disparities from 400 to 100 seconds of arc.

Precautions
- Appropriate tests should be selected for the age and level of cooperation of the patient.

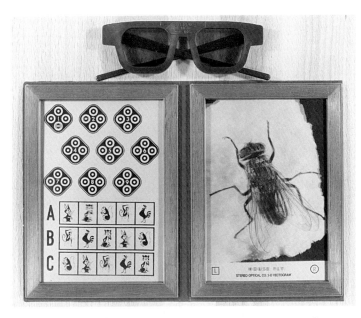

Fig. 7.6   *Titmus fly and Wirt circles.*

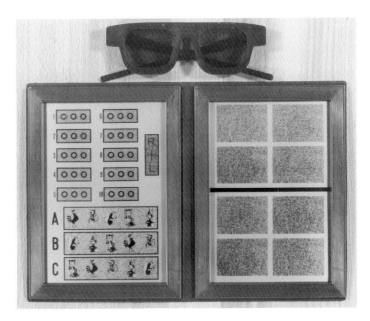

Fig. 7.7   *Random dot (right) and Wirt circles (left).*

- The correct working distance should be used to ensure that the disparity levels achieved are accurate.

Key points
- Good illumination is required.
- Sufficient presentation time is needed to allow appreciation of the disparity.

- Large disparity targets detect the presence of normal and anomalous BSV. Stereoacuity of 40 seconds of arc or better indicates bifoveal BSV and a well compensated binocular status.
- Poorly compensated deviations and amblyopia will result in poor or absent depth perception.
- Our method of choice is the TNO test provided that sufficient cooperation is present.
- A demonstrable level of stereoacuity in the presence of a heterotropia is diagnostic of abnormal retinal correspondence (ARC).

Tests to assess the state of retinal correspondence

Two types of retinal correspondence exist where retinal areas of either eye correspond in binocular viewing.

- *Normal retinal correspondence (NRC)* – the fovea of one eye has a common visual direction with the fovea of the other eye. Retinal points nasal to one fovea correspond to those temporal to the other fovea. The objective angle of deviation equals the subjective angle.
- *Abnormal retinal correspondence (ARC)* – the fovea of one eye has a common visual direction with an extrafoveal point. All other retinal points are similarly changed and correspond. The objective angle is larger than the subjective angle, the difference equating to the angle of anomaly. ARC is harmonious when the objective angle equals the angle of anomaly.

Modified Mallett (large) OXO test

The near Mallett unit can be used to prove the existence of ARC in the presence of a small-angle deviation in a similar way to Bagolini lenses.

Method

- With optimum refractive correction and polarizing filters in place, the patient should be asked to view the standard OXO and vertical green markers on the near Mallett unit, which are used in the determination of horizontal fixation disparity.
- In the presence of a small-angle deviation, the green marker that corresponds to the deviating eye will not be seen because of the presence of a small suppression scotoma.
- The patient should then be instructed to fix the larger OXO in the top left-hand corner of all modern near Mallett units.
- If, in the presence of a small-angle deviation, both the green markers are seen, ARC must be present in the deviating eye. This occurs because the green markers on the large OXO are much larger than the suppression scotomas associated with ARC.
- If only older Mallett units without the larger OXO are available, the distance Mallett unit viewed at 1.5 m can be used.

Bagolini lenses

This is a minimally dissociative test available in a reversible lorgnette (Fig. 7.8) or trial frame form (Fig. 7.9). Each plano glass lens has fine parallel striations inscribed on to the surface. A spotlight is converted into a line image seen at 90° to the striations.

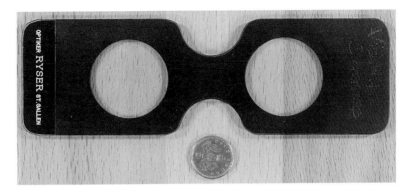

Fig. 7.8 *Bagolini lenses lorgnette.*

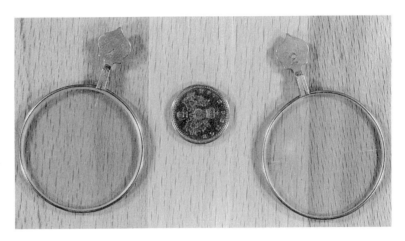

Fig. 7.9 *Bagolini lenses trial frame form.*

Method

With any refractive correction in situ, the patient is asked to fixate a spotlight at 6 m under normal lighting conditions and the lenses are placed in front of both eyes if the deviation alternates, but only in front of the deviating eye if the deviation is unilateral. The patient is asked how many spotlights are seen, then the amount and exact position of the lines. Repeat for 33 cm.

Possible results (Fig. 7.10)

- A symmetrical cross centred on the spotlight (assuming an alternating deviation) indicates BSV or harmonious ARC. Differentiation can be made using the cover test, which would normally elicit a small heterotropia if correspondence was abnormal.
- A gap in one of the lines relates to a foveal suppression scotoma (rarely reported by patients).
- Displaced lines (with or without appreciation of two lights) indicates heterotropia with NRC. Confirmation can be made by adding

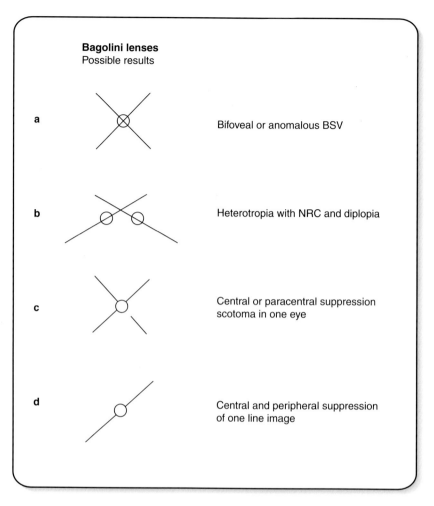

Fig. 7.10 *Possible results with Bagolini lenses. (a) Bifoveal or anomalous BSV. (b) Heterotropia with NRC and diplopia. (c) Central or paracentral suppression scotoma in one eye. (d) Central and peripheral suppression of one line image.*

prism strength equal to the angle of deviation. A symmetrical cross will be produced in NRC, but crossed projection in an esotropic patient with ARC.
- One spotlight and one line image indicates central and peripheral suppression.

Key point

Appreciation of the **X** in the presence of a heterotropia is diagnostic of a small-angle deviation with ARC or of a microtropia with ARC or NRC.

Worth's four lights

The test consists of four illuminated circles on a black or grey background: one red, one white and two green. When viewed through complementary red and green filters, the white light is common to both eyes and therefore acts as a stimulus to fusion. The red and white lights are seen through the red filter, and the green and white lights through the green filter (Fig. 7.11). The test is available in forms for use at 6 m and 33 cm.

Method

- The red filter is usually placed in front of the right eye and the green filter in front of the left eye.
- Viewing the test at 6 m, the patient is asked how many lights of each colour are seen.
- The test can be repeated for 33 cm, but the results are not generally thought to be reliable.

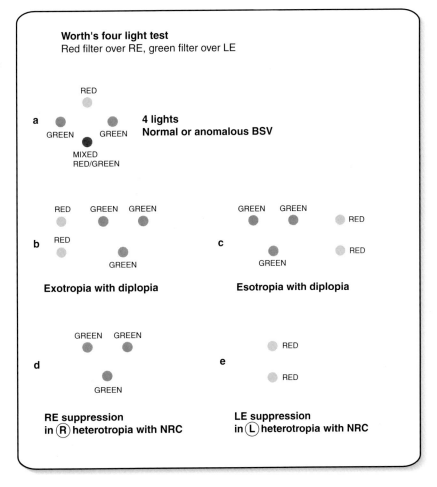

Fig. 7.11 *Worth's four lights test, with red filter over right eye and green filter over left eye.*

Possible results

Four lights

BSV – the lower circle is often seen as an alternation of red and green, or may be the colour seen by the dominant eye. The cover test can differentiate NRC (heterotropia absent) from harmonious ARC (heterotropia present).

Five lights

Heterotropia with diplopia - NRC is present if the lights are superimposed to situation 1 with a prism equal in strength to the angle of deviation.

Two or three lights

Suppression – only one colour will be seen if suppression is unilateral, or the colours will alternate if suppression is alternating.

Use of prisms to assess retinal correspondence

Principle

In horizontal heterotropia, a vertical prism will displace an image on to the non-suppressed retina and the patient will recognize diplopia. The horizontal measurement of the vertically diplopic images determines whether correspondence is normal or abnormal.

Equipment

- Vertical and horizontal prisms.
- Spotlight at 6 m.

Method

- The patient fixates a spotlight at 6 m.
- A 10Δ vertical prism is placed in front of one eye.
- The patient is asked to describe the position of the two lights (recognition of diplopia can be facilitated by placing a coloured filter in front of one eye).

Results

- Either a horizontal prism of strength equal to the angle of deviation will place the images directly vertical to one another, denoting NRC; or
- A prism strength equal to the angle of deviation will change the projection from uncrossed to crossed diplopia in esotropia and from crossed to uncrossed in exotropia, denoting ARC.

8 Oculomotility testing

Introduction

The main reasons for carrying out oculomotility testing are to elicit the extent and quality of movement of each eye, to determine the presence of comitancy or incomitancy and whether any change in the size of the deviation is due to decompensation of a heterophoria or a muscle defect, and to establish the integrity of the ocular movement systems and their neural pathways.

Method

- Use a spotlight positioned in the primary position of gaze at 50 cm from the patient.
- Always remove the patient's glasses for the following reasons:
  - Frames and the increase in effective power at the lens periphery limit the field of view.
  - Prismatic effects may be induced in the lens periphery.
  - Reflection of the spotlight on the lenses can confuse interpretation of the findings.
  - The spotlight can be seen without glasses even by those with high refractive error.
- Give clear instructions to the patient, such as:
  - to keep the head straight throughout testing
  - to report whether, at any point, the patient appreciates diplopia (horizontal, vertical, torsional or a combination) and in which position it is greatest
  - to report whether there is any discomfort or pain during testing.
- Perform the alternate cover test in the primary position, comparing primary and secondary angles of deviation in heterotropia.
- Move the spotlight slowly and smoothly from the primary position each time into the extremes of gaze, ensuring that the corneal reflections are present on each eye.
- An audible or colourful fixation target may need to be used instead of, or in combination with, a spotlight for young children.
- Test horizontal versions and look for the following:
  - updrift or downdrift of either eye
  - underaction or overaction of extraocular muscles
  - limitation (restriction of movement)
  - changes in the size of the palpebral aperture
  - changes in pupil size
  - changes in globe position.
- Repeat the alternate cover test in the extreme positions of gaze. The size of the dissociated deviation will increase in the direction of the affected muscle(s). If any defect is found on versions, ductions should

be assessed, i.e. in the primary position occlude the fixing eye and observe the position of the corneal reflection as the spotlight is moved into the extreme position of gaze. There are two possible results:

— The eye takes up fixation of the light, the corneal reflection remains central for the whole excursion and the movement is full. This indicates an underaction of the muscle that acts maximally in this position of gaze.

— The eye takes up fixation for part of the excursion followed by cessation of movement and the corneal reflection is no longer central. This indicates a limitation (restriction) of movement.

- Test direct elevation and observe for:
  — underaction, overaction and limitation
  — globe changes
  — signs of lid or extraocular muscle fatigue by testing sustained elevation (Simpson's test).

- When testing direct depression, first perform without raising the upper lids so that any associated anomalies of lid movement can be seen.

Alphabet patterns

- The alternate cover test in direct elevation and depression is compared to elicit the presence of an A or V pattern, i.e. a change in the horizontal angle of deviation (other patterns can exist, such as Y or X).

- Using the prism cover test, an A pattern is diagnosed if there is a difference of 10Δ or more between direct elevation and depression.

- V patterns are diagnosed if there is a difference of 15Δ or more – this accounts for the physiological V pattern of approximately 5Δ.

- Patterns can be thought of as physiological incomitant deviations and are due to imbalances between the vertically acting muscles that produce horizontal changes from their secondary muscle actions (Fig. 8.1), for example the superior rectus.

- The A or V pattern is termed eso or exo according to the deviation found using an alternate cover test in the primary position of gaze (see Patient II on the CD-ROM).

Oblique positions

- Test elevated positions first to compare directly the same synergistic pairs of muscles in right and left gaze followed by the depressed positions and observe for:
  — underaction, overaction or limitation
  — changes in globe position
  — changes in lid position or lid movement.

Hess charts

These provide an aid to the diagnosis, measurement and monitoring of ocular motility defects.

Principle

Two main types of screen are in use and both are based on:

- Foveal projection – patients must demonstrate normal correspondence and no suppression
- Hering's and Sherrington's laws of innervation
- Dissociation via complementary colours or a mirror.

Hess screen

- This consists of a black or grey tangent screen (Fig. 8.2).
- Dissociation is achieved by using red and green filters with the red filter in front of the fixing eye.

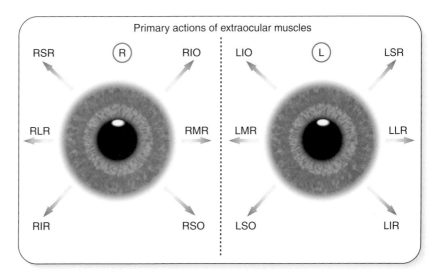

Fig. 8.1 *Oculomotility. Arrows show primary actions of extraocular muscles. Dotted line: moving a pen torch in the vertical midline will test secondary actions and detect alphabet patterns. RSR = right superior rectus, RIO = right inferior oblique, RMR = right medial rectus, RSO = right superior oblique, RIR = right inferior rectus, RLR = right lateral rectus, LIO = left inferior oblique, LSR = left superior rectus, LLR = left lateral rectus, LIR = left inferior rectus, LSO = left superior oblique and LMR = left medial rectus.*

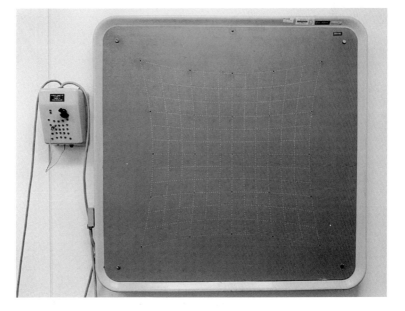

Fig. 8.2 *Hess tangent screen.*

- The chart is divided by red lines into 10° sections extending out to 30° from fixation.
- The fixating eye sees a tangent pattern with red lights and the non-fixating eye sees a green light projected on to the screen via a torch held by the patient 50 cm away.
- The discrepancy between the two colours on the screen is plotted on a paper chart to record the extent of the deviation.
- The test is repeated by fixating with the other eye to compare primary and secondary angles of deviation.
- A computerized desktop version is available.

Lees screen
- This consists of two internally illuminated opaque screens positioned at 90° to each other with black tangent grids marked on their back surfaces (Fig. 8.3). Each square subtends 5° at the testing distance of 50 cm. Black dots are positioned at intervals of 15° and 30°, giving an inner and outer field plot.
- A double-sided plane mirror positioned at 45° to the screens achieves dissociation.
- The fixating eye views the illuminated screen directly and the other views the non-illuminated second screen via the mirror.
- The examiner uses a pointer to indicate the dot to be fixated and the patient responds by placing their pointer on the indicated dot on the non-illuminated screen.
- This screen is briefly illuminated and the position of the dot is recorded on the chart.
- When all of the dots have been plotted, the patient is turned through 90° to repeat the test fixating with the other eye.

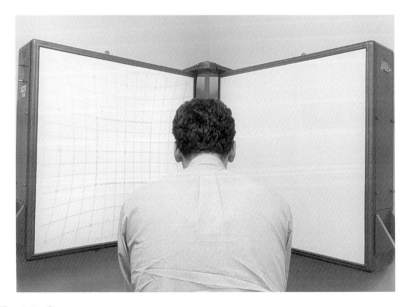

Fig. 8.3 *Lees screen.*

Interpretation

Position

- Use of foveal projection produces displacement of the field in the direction of the deviation (e.g. higher in a hyperdeviation).
- The position of the central dot in each field indicates the deviation in the primary position, fixing with the right eye on the left chart and with the left eye on the right chart.

Size

- In accordance with Hering's law of equal innervation, the smaller field (plotted with the more mobile eye fixating) belongs to the eye with the primary ocular motility defect.
- Underaction is denoted by inward displacement of the dots, and overaction by outward displacement.
- A narrow field in opposing directions indicates a mechanical restriction of movement.
- Fields of equal size denote development of muscle sequelae and a long-standing deviation.
- See CD Patients 7 and 13 for examples of Hess charts.

Shape

- Slanting fields indicate A and V patterns.

Key point

Both types of screen can be adapted to assess torsion by using linear targets instead of the dots.

Compensatory head postures

A compensatory head posture (CHP) exists when there is a deviation of the head from the primary position. It may be present as a mechanism for overcoming an ocular abnormality or for non-ocular reasons.

A CHP can have three components, present either singly or in a combination of:

- face turn to the right or left side
- head tilt to the right or left shoulder
- chin elevation or depression.

Only ocular reasons for a CHP are discussed here.

Ocular head postures

Reasons:

- diplopia
- limitation of ocular movement
- defective visual function
- discomfort or pain in one or more gaze positions.

CHP in paralytic strabismus

Reasons:

- To place the eyes in a position of least deviation to enable the maintenance or development of BSV
- To centralize the field of binocular fixation
- To obtain foveal fixation when movement of the eye is restricted
- To avoid looking into an area of gaze where there is discomfort or pain.

Face turn

- To place the eyes away from the field of primary action of the palsied muscle into the position of least deviation (e.g. face turn to the left in left VI nerve palsy).

Head tilt

- Vertical deviations – the head is tilted to the side of the hypodeviated eye. This lowers the higher image produced by the deviated eye and the two images can then be fused (e.g. right head tilt in right hypotropia).
- Torsional deviations – in 'normals' when the head is tilted to the right shoulder, the right eye intorts and the left eye extorts to maintain binocular single vision. However, when there is a vertical deviation, due for example, to a right IV nerve palsy, the right eye is already extorted, so to compensate the head is tilted to the left shoulder.
- See patient 13 on CD.

Chin elevation or depression

Reasons:

- To place the eyes away from the main field of action of the palsied muscle (e.g. chin depression in a IV nerve palsy)
- To place the eyes in a position of least deviation where binocular single vision can be maintained (e.g. chin elevation in a Y exo pattern)
- To avoid an area of discomfort (e.g. chin elevation in patients with dysthyroid eye disease; chin elevation in patients with a blow-out fracture).

CHP in defective visual function

Reason:

- To place the eyes in a position where a clearer image can be obtained.

Nystagmus

- Congenital – an eccentric null zone can be centralized by adopting a face turn.
- Latent – in patients with infantile esotropia and alternating fixation, a face turn may be adopted to adduct the fixing eye in an attempt to induce convergence and reduce the nystagmoid eye movements.

Foveal fixation

A large restriction of ocular movement in the fixing eye may necessitate a CHP to achieve normal fixation.

Visual field defects

Patients with visual field defects may adopt a face turn or a chin elevation or depression to place the eyes away from the area of visual loss (e.g. left face turn in left homonymous hemianopia).

Incorrect refractive correction

If spectacles have been incorrectly prescribed or fitted, or if the refractive error changes, both the visual acuity and patient comfort may be improved by adopting a CHP.

Long-standing CHP

A reduction in the size of components of a CHP can occur with the development of comitance (e.g. end-stage muscle sequelae in a IV nerve palsy usually eliminate the need for chin depression), extension of the fusion amplitude with time, or improvement in ocular motility.

Clinical examination

CHPs can vary in their components and size between distance and near fixation. Assessment should be made by asking the patient to fixate a detailed target at both distances:

- Initially observe for the presence of any facial asymmetry that may produce a pseudo-CHP.
- Determine the components of the CHP and note the position into which the eyes have been placed.
- Observe the patient's head position when testing uniocular and binocular visual acuity.
- A cover test should be performed both with and without the CHP. This will determine whether the CHP has been adopted for ocular or non-ocular reasons. A deviation will not increase in magnitude without the CHP if the CHP has non-ocular origins.

Key point

Previous photographs may indicate the duration of the CHP and help to diagnose the aetiology of the ocular abnormality.

Congenital and acquired incomitant deviations (Table 8.1)

Aetiology and investigation

The cause of any palsy must be investigated to eliminate any sight- or life-threatening conditions, although when the palsy is long-standing the patient may have been investigated previously and will often know the cause. Changes to a long-standing condition may need to be re-investigated. These costly and possibly unpleasant tests are unnecessary in patients with a congenital palsy that has already been investigated.

Observation

In acquired palsies, time must be allowed for the development of muscle sequelae and recovery – approximately 6 months, or longer if the deviation is changing. Congenital palsies can be treated without delay.

Key points

It is important to take a detailed case history, with particular reference to the mode of onset of diplopia and the presence of any compensatory mechanisms the patient may have adopted.

The development of comitance is not always a reliable sign of a long-standing deviation. In our experience, all comitant palsies are congenital or long-standing, but not all congenital or long-standing palsies are comitant.

The presence of CHP seen on old photographs is diagnostic of long duration if compatible with the type of palsy seen when examined.

Neurogenic and mechanical incomitant deviations

See Table 8.2.

Table 8.1 *Differential diagnosis of congenital and acquired incomitant deviations*

	Congenital	Acquired
History	• Diplopia common, but onset of diplopia vague and intermittent • Indefinite symptoms of blurring or headaches due to effort to control • Chance discovery • Child may attend due to strabismus or CHP • Duration uncertain	• Diplopia invariable • Exact onset of diplopia known and patient may be aware of the cause
Head position	• Patient and family often unaware of CHP • CHP may be slight in comparison to deviation; scoliosis may be present in presence of a head tilt • Facial asymmetry common • Change in chin position may not be present if palsy is comitant • CHP often seen on old photograph	• Patient aware of CHP • Often uncomfortable to maintain • May be marked, even with slight deviation • Chin elevation or depression an obvious feature in a vertical palsy
Ocular movement or concomitance	• Muscle sequelae are usually well developed, leading to relative concomitance • Hess chart shows approximately equally sized fields; primary and secondary underactions roughly equal • Difficult to diagnose primarily affected muscles	• Overaction of contralateral synergist present, but other muscle sequelae have not developed • Secondary deviation larger than primary; field of affected eye much smaller on Hess chart than that of non-affected eye
Fusion amplitude	• Patients with congenital vertical palsies usually have a large vertical fusion range of 10∆ or more; field of BSV quite large	• Normal fusion range; exceptions are patients with gradual onset or long duration of limitations of movement (e.g. dysthyroid eye disease)
Suppression	• May be present, but usually intermittent	• Suppression rarely occurs, except in children or older patients (especially those with poor vision)
Torsion	• Less common in IV nerve palsies owing to spread of comitance	• Usual in IV nerve palsy, especially when bilateral

CHP, compensatory head posture; BSV, binocular single vision.

Table 8.2 *Differential diagnosis of neurogenic and mechanical incomitant deviations (Continued on p. 78)*

	Neurogenic	Mechanical
History	• May have history of systemic or neurological disease • Cause may be unknown • Onset may be gradual (e.g. decompensation of long-standing IV nerve palsy) or sudden (e.g. total III nerve palsy)	• Aetiology: injury to orbit or muscles, inflammation in orbit or muscles, congenital conditions, orbital tumour or pseudo-tumour • Sudden onset if due to trauma; may be more gradual if inflammatory • No neurological signs, unless patient has had associated head injury
Symptoms	• Usually diplopia, gradual or sudden onset • Possibly of long duration if congenital	• Diplopia in acquired cases • In congenital conditions (e.g. Duane's or Brown's syndrome) diplopia is less common (often due to early development of CHP) • May not be present in primary position • Often reverses (e.g. up to down gaze) • Pain on movement
Signs CHP	• May be one or a combination of face turn, head tilt and chin depression or elevation • Chin depression or elevation tends to reduce with the development of muscle sequelae	• Tilt uncommon, because torsion unlikely • CHP slight compared with extent of limitation • CHP may be present to avoid pain or discomfort

Other	• Facial asymmetry in congenital vertical palsies	• Possible displacement of globe:
		  —exophthalmos (e.g. orbital space-occupying lesion, dysthyroid eye disease)
		  —enophthalmos (e.g. orbital blow-out fracture)
		  —upward or downward displacement of the globe in a facial fracture

Table 8.2 *Differential diagnosis of neurogenic and mechanical incomitant deviations—Continued*

	Neurogenic	Mechanical
		• Bruising or scarring in facial area and injuries to trochlear or infraorbital area
		• Possible lid changes (e.g. narrowing palpebral aperture on adduction in Duane's retraction syndrome, lid retraction in dysthyroid eye disease)
Diplopia	• Follows recognizable pattern for palsy	• Diplopia may reverse due to mechanical restriction of the muscle or its surrounding tissue (e.g. L/R on elevation, R/L on depression)
	• May have torsional diplopia depending on muscles affected and duration (common in superior oblique palsy)	• May have very long, narrow 'squashed' BSV field if limitations are in two opposing directions
		• Torsional diplopia less likely
Ophthalmological investigations		
Forced duction test	Negative (normal)	Positive (abnormal)
IOP measurement	No variation with position of gaze	Rise in IOP in direction of maximum limitation if tethered orbital tissue or infiltrated extraocular muscles apply pressure on globe
Electromyography	Depends on muscle innervation (e.g. may be silent in paralysis)	Electromyogram shows normal firing pattern
Saccadic velocity	Saccadic velocity and amplitude significantly reduced	Saccadic velocity within normal limits until point of mechanical tethering is reached, but amplitude is reduced

CHP, compensatory head posture; BSV, binocular single vision; IOP, intraocular pressure; L, left; R, right.

Routines

Introduction

This chapter describes three typical routines that we have found useful in our clinical practice when examining patients for the first time. Follow-up appointments may include all or just a selection of these tests, depending on the individual case. None of these routines is meant to be prescriptive and the tests are probably not exhaustive. Also, the exact nature of an evaluation of binocular vision will depend on whether there are any presenting symptoms or signs and on the cooperation and ability of the patient. The order in which tests are carried out may be varied according to personal preference.

Typical routine for a child aged less than 1 year

This routine is also applicable for any patient who is not capable of communicating with the practitioner.
- History and symptoms obtained from attending carer
- Observe patient, looking for gross strabismus, CHP, ptosis, anisocoria, manifest nystagmus
- Hirschberg's corneal reflexes
- Brückner test
- Monocular visual acuity using Cardiff acuity cards or Keeler acuity cards
- Cover test, distance and near, using small detailed targets likely to be of interest to the patient
- Oculomotility using a target likely to be of interest and not necessarily a pen torch, looking for underactions, overactions, limitations, alphabet patterns or tendencies, lid changes and globe changes
- 10Δ base-out fusional vergence test
- Retinoscopy using the near fixation technique or cycloplegia
- Stereoacuity using Lang I, and Lang II using preferential looking technique
- Direct ophthalmoscopy or modified monocular or head-mounted indirect ophthalmoscopy.

Typical routine for a young child (e.g. 4 years old)

- History and symptoms obtained mainly from attending carer
- Observe patient, looking for gross strabismus, associated head posture, ptosis, anisocoria or manifest latent nystagmus
- Hirschberg's corneal reflexes
- Brückner test
- Monocular distance visual acuity using Keeler logMAR uncrowded or crowded cards with matching card where necessary
- Near visual acuity using logMAR near letter acuity card, Maclure cards or the Faculty of Ophthalmologists' reading acuity cards (may need to use letters rather than words)

- Cover test, distance and near, using small detailed targets likely to be of interest to the patient
- Oculomotility using a target likely to be of interest and not necessarily a pen torch; conduct alternate cover test in nine positions of gaze and look for underactions, overactions, limitations, alphabet patterns and tendencies, lid changes and globe changes
- 20∆ base-out fusional vergence test
- Retinoscopy using the distance static or near fixation technique or cycloplegia
- Stereoacuity using Titmus–Wirt circles or the TNO test
- Direct ophthalmoscopy or modified monocular or head-mounted indirect ophthalmoscopy.

Typical routine for an older child or adult

- History and symptoms usually obtained from the patient
- Observe patient, looking for gross strabismus, CHP, ptosis, anisocoria, manifest nystagmus
- Monocular and binocular distance and near visual acuity using Snellen or logMAR chart and a near visual acuity or reading acuity chart
- Oculomotility using a pen torch and conducting an alternate cover test in nine positions of gaze, looking for underactions, overactions, limitations, alphabet patterns, lid changes, globe changes, pain on movement
- Retinoscopy distance static technique
- Subjective refraction
- Colour vision test
- Direct ophthalmoscopy.

Heterophoria or microtropia

- The distance unilateral cover–uncover test and the alternating cover test should be conducted using a small letter target. For presbyopes the near cover test should be conducted using a spotlight target only, and both a letter target and a light for pre-presbyopes.
- Prism cover test at distance using a small letter target, and at near using a small letter target and a light
- Maddox rod at distance to look for small vertical deviations
- Maddox wing at near to look for small vertical and cyclodeviations
- Near point of convergence
- Monocular and binocular amplitudes of accommodation
- Fusional vergence reserves
- Aligning prism or sphere at distance and near
- Foveal suppression test in heterophoria
- Eccentric fixation in microtropia
- Presence of ARC using Bagolini lenses or standard and large OXO targets on near Mallett unit
- Depth of ARC using Bagolini lenses and Sbiza bar or neutral density filters in front of deviating eye
- Stereoacuity Titmus–Wirt circles or TNO test
- AC/A ratio.

Heterotropia

- Unilateral cover test at distance using a small letter target, and using a small letter target and a spotlight at near for pre-presbyopes and a spotlight for presbyopes

- Simultaneous prism cover test at distance using a small letter target, and a small letter target and a spotlight at near (when appropriate)
- Monocular and binocular amplitudes of accommodation for pre-presbyopes
- Depth of suppression (when strabismus is present without diplopia) using Bagolini lenses and Sbiza bar or neutral density filter in front of the non-deviating eye
- Lees screen or Hess screen.

The following is a list of questions, many of which have been used in past professional qualifying examinations (PQEs) for optometrists. We have provided this to give the reader a flavour of the typical questions asked. The list is not prescriptive or exhaustive. Also, we have deliberately not provided the answers as we believe that learning is best achieved through a combination of book work, practice of techniques and discussions with supervisors, optometrists and other eye care specialists.

1. What is amblyopia and how would you classify it?
2. Explain how you would differentiate strabismic and anisometropic amblyopia.
3. Discuss in general terms how to interpret a Lees or Hess screen plot to identify incomitancy.
4. What factors influence the development of ARC in people with strabismus?
5. Describe how you would investigate a strabismic patient to determine their sensory status.
6. How would you treat a strabismic amblyope? Give three methods in the order in which they might be applied.
7. What do you understand by the terms convergence insufficiency and divergence excess?
8. Indicate the methods for using the Mallett unit to detect ARC and uncompensated heterophoria.
9. Discuss the role of surgery in the management of strabismus.
10. Describe the clinical features of amblyopia of arrest, V syndrome, Duane's retraction syndrome, and harmonious ARC.
11. Indicate the possible courses of management for the following: a young myope with divergence excess; a marked hypermetropic anisometrope with convergent strabismus and amblyopia; a teenager with asthenopic symptoms and convergence insufficiency; a presbyope with increasing exophoria becoming uncompensated.
12. A 5-year-old child presents for an eye examination and, on initial examination, appears to have a subjective refraction of R+2.00 L+2.00. However, you detected R and L +4.00 on retinoscopy. What will you do next? What will you then prescribe? What are your instructions to the carers?
13. What stereoacuity test do you use? What are its drawbacks?

83

14. You see a 7-year-old with a visual acuity of R6/6 L6/18 who is fully corrected and wearing glasses all the time. Discuss your options for treatment. *Patch amb eye 5hrs/day; 1wk; retun — imp. continue - nothing op poss if*

ambyope, Tropia? Pathology?

15. What is internuclear ophthalmoplegia and where does it occur in the brainstem?

16. What is optokinetic nystagmus?

17. What causes congenital nystagmus?

18. What is the level of visual acuity at birth?

19. How would you measure visual acuity in a child aged (a) less than 2 years and (b) more than 2 years?

20. Draw or explain the insertion of the superior oblique. What action does it have?

21. What is commonly associated with a superior rectus paresis? Why is this? *SR TO levator*

22. Explain the concept of Panum's areas.

23. What is fixation disparity?

24. Which is more accurate, accommodation or convergence? Which develops first and at what ages do they develop?

25. A 7-year-old child presents with no current spectacles. Cover test reveals a 20Δ alternating exotropia at distance, 15Δ exophoria at near, accommodative amplitude of 18.00DS, and near point of convergence (NPC) of 6 cm. How would you investigate and treat? *llcpm monoc; 6 c 8m binoc.*

Should have no amblyopia ? BV? Stereo? Amp of accom too low for 7 you Exercises accom rod/flipper tracing, 100's + 1000's

26. Why is there an increased prevalence of strabismus in children at 2 years of age?

27. Why does strabismus sometimes occur after measles?

28. A 70-year-old patient reports sudden-onset diplopia. What questions should you ask?

29. A patient presents with 20Δ esotropia at distance, 4Δ esophoria at near. What are the possible causes? Which non-binocular vision test would you conduct? What is your course of action?

30. A 20-year-old patient has R6/6 L6/6, accommodative amplitude right and left 18.00DS, no refractive error right and left, cover test no deviation at distance, cover test at near 8Δ esophoria. What symptoms would you expect? What would be your line of management? *?*

31. How would you determine whether the 8Δ esophoria is a problem to the patient?

32. Which nerves innervate the extraocular muscles?

33. Describe the pathway of the IV nerve.

34. Describe the pathway of the VI nerve.

35. Describe the pathway of the III nerve.

36. What is the effect of a partial III nerve lesion?

37. What would you see with a IV nerve defect?

38. What are common causes of lesions of the III, IV and VI nerves?

39. What are the different components of the binocular vision system and how are they assessed clinically?

40. Your patient has a near decompensating exophoria. How would you assess this patient and what would be your management?

Watch out for eccentric viewing +ecc. fixat as becomes more ingrained if fixat disparity not treated. exercises, full Rx @ near + poss inc. -ve; prisms Assess the fusion reserve (Base out); NPC; amp. accom; H+S; age?

[Handwritten at top: observe Px, H+S, CT, Hirschberg, Dist acuity @ 1m - motility targets OPHTHAL crowded D+N matching letters. Titmus: stereopsis, cyclo.]

41. How would you measure the vision of a 3-year-old child?

42. What are the positive fusional reserves? What is their magnitude? *[handwritten: ability to converge blur/break/recovery neg 35-40 BO dist 15-20 BO]*

43. What is an associated phoria?

44. You have diagnosed a 3-year-old child as having a fully accommodative strabismus. How would you manage this patient? *[handwritten: gls/CL]*

45. What problems might partial refractive correction cause in this patient? *[handwritten: tropia due to near demands, AC/A ratio]*

46. How do you know whether a patient's phoria is decompensating? *[handwritten: mallet, aesthopia]*

47. How would you investigate a patient who complains of diplopia when hanging clothes on a washing line?

48. How would you assess a 2-year-old child?

49. Draw the muscle insertions and the centre of rotation of the eye.

50. What problems would someone with a frontal bone blow-out have? *[handwritten: Dip esp vert move]*

51. Why is it important to have two eyes? *[handwritten: BV, stereopsis, redundancy, dist judg]*

52. Describe how the age of the patient determines which stereoacuity test is the most appropriate to use. *[handwritten: concrete, sit still, easy to understand, gross stereo if - young.]*

53. How would you modify your routine for a child?

54. How would you measure NPC? What would be a normal result? *[handwritten: RAF rule 10cm]*

[handwritten diagram on left margin with L and R markings]

55. What is physiological diplopia? How do crossed and uncrossed physiological diplopia differ? *[handwritten: crossed, diplop target nearer temporal]*

56. Why is it more serious to have a convergent strabismus than a divergent one? *[handwritten: intra = tumour, vas. accident]*

57. What are gaze palsies and what is their significance?

58. What are Brown's and Duane's syndromes? *[handwritten: SO tendon restrict; RMR + LR both constrict]*

59. What features would you look for on a Hess chart in order to determine whether an incomitant deviation was due to a muscle palsy or a muscle restriction? *[handwritten: - narrow field opposing direct -]*

[handwritten left margin: iger = palsied eye]

60. What is the difference between a muscle palsy and a muscle paralysis?

61. An underaction of which muscle is most likely to result in a problem with reading? *[handwritten: iris; ciliary; MR]*

62. How would you manage a patient with frontal headaches and a receded near point of convergence? *[handwritten: motility, diplop/pathology?; exercise, vergence control, + lenses]*

63. How can small modifications of the spherical refractive correction be used for symptomatic patients? *[handwritten: inc, + for nr. work; NPC probs,]*

64. How can small prisms incorporated into a refractive correction be used for symptomatic patients? *[handwritten: lab off, stick on,]*

65. How would you determine what amount of prism to use in this case? *[handwritten: Mallett]*

66. What do you understand by the term *prism adaptation*? *[handwritten: wear prism 5mins read ee, alt. CT w. prism, + iger prism needed has adapted]*

67. What is Sheard's criterion?

68. What is Percival's criterion?

69. What does the Lang II stereoacuity test have as a target that can be seen monocularly? *[handwritten star]*

70. What is the range in seconds of arc of the following stereoacuity tests: Lang I, Lang II, Titmus/Wirt, TNO, and Frisby? *[handwritten: 1200➔550", 3000➔100" 480➔15"]*

71. At what age does stereoacuity start to develop and when is it fully developed?
72. What is the refractive error of a newborn child most likely to be?
73. What do you understand by the term emmetropisation?
74. If a 4-year-old child presented with –1.00DC with the rule astigmatism, what would be your management?
75. Would you correct a 4-year-old with right and left +2.00DS? What other factors would you take into account?
76. What is meant by the AC/A ratio? How would you measure it? What is considered to be a normal value?
77. What would you expect to see on a near cover test for a child wearing their full distance refractive correction if they have an AC/A ratio of 7:1?
78. How would you manage a person with convergence excess?
79. What is the difference between convergence insufficiency and a convergence weakness exophoria?
80. What exercises would you recommend to a patient with convergence insufficiency? How often and for how long should they carry out these exercises? When would you review them?
81. What are free space stereograms? Give an example.
82. How would you attempt to manage divergence insufficiency?
83. What do you understand by the term *preferential looking*?
84. Why do VEP techniques produce higher visual acuities values at a younger age than techniques involving preferential looking?
85. Describe a preferential looking test you are familiar with.
86. How do you know when you have reached the end point with this test?
87. What would you expect the visual acuity to be for a 2-year-old with this test?
88. A 20-year-old patient presents complaining of occipital headaches and you find right and left +0.75DS. How would you manage this patient?
89. A mother presents with her 4-year-old child and mentions that she often sees the child's right eye turn in. You carry out all the necessary tests but cannot detect any deviation. What is your management?
90. When would you use a cycloplegic? What is your drug of choice?
91. Are there are any adverse reactions associated with this drug?
92. What type of nerve palsy is most commonly associated with diabetes?
93. Why do people with dysthyroid eye disease often have problems looking up?
94. Which extraocular muscles would be affected by a superior branch III nerve palsy?
95. Which extraocular muscles would be affected by an inferior branch III nerve palsy?

96. What is a common cause of a III nerve palsy?
97. Why is the VI nerve susceptible to trauma?
98. Why is the IV nerve susceptible to trauma?
99. How would you manage a patient with Brown's syndrome?
100. How would you manage a patient with Duane's syndrome?

Eccentric fixat⁻ - Posit⁻ where amblyopic fixes
when gd eye covered (not practed fixat⁻ pt)

11   Video clips on the CD-ROM

Demonstration of cover test technique	This video clip demonstrates the technique we recommend when carrying out a cover–uncover and an alternating cover test (p. 21–35).
Patient 1	This patient has a fully accommodative alternating esotropia. The key to diagnosing this condition is to compare the near cover test with and without glasses in place. If the patient doesn't wear glasses then a near cover test movement that is larger to a letter target than to a light target is highly suggestive of at least an accommodative element to the deviation (p. 24).
Patient 2	This patient has Duane's retraction syndrome Type A. The key to making this diagnosis is by good observation and noting the presence of a compensatory head posture (CHP) and to conduct a thorough oculomotility test looking out for any globe retraction (p. 73–75).
Patient 3	This patient has a right VI nerve palsy and a right partial ptosis. This diagnosis can be made using a combination of observation (p. 75), cover testing (p. 21–34) and oculomotility testing (p. 69).
Patient 4	This patient has a consecutive left exotropia post left medial rectus recession and right lateral rectus resection, with dissociated vertical divergence. The diagnosis can be made by conducting a cover test and an oculomotility test.
Patient 5	This patient has right Brown's syndrome. A key point is observing the extreme difficulty the patient has in elevation during oculomotility testing (p. 69).
Patient 6	This patient has dysthyroid eye disease. Observation will reveal left proptosis and restricted eye movements during oculomotility testing (p. 76).
Patient 7	This patient has a right III nerve palsy that is recovering. This diagnosis is best made using alternate cover testing in all nine positions of gaze during oculomotility testing (p. 28).
Patient 8	This patient has a fully accommodative left to alternating esotropia. As with patient 1 the key to this diagnosis is to conduct a cover test at near with and without glasses (p. 24–25). A larger deviation without glasses is very suggestive of an accommodative element.

Patient 9

This patient has a residual intermittent right distance exotropia (simulated), following right lateral rectus recession and medial rectus resection. The diagnosis can be made using the cover test. A slightly reduced near point of convergence as measured with an RAF rule (p. 39) assists in the decision-making process.

Patient 10

This patient has a large right esotropia and DVD. The presence of a right esotropia is obvious but it can be confirmed using Hirschberg's test and unilateral cover-uncover of the left eye.

Patient 11

This patient has congenital partial right ptosis and right micro-esotropia. A combination of observation of a right ptosis and forehead skin crease along with cover and alternate cover testing will help make this diagnosis.

Patient 12

This patient has an exophoria and a V exo pattern. Alternate cover testing in the primary, depressed and elevated positions of gaze is the key to this diagnosis (p. 30).

Patient 13

This patient has a long-standing right IV nerve palsy with compensatory left head tilt (p. 74). Observation of the CHP, and alternate cover testing with oculomotility testing are the keys to making this diagnosis.

Index